# HIP, HIP, HOORAY!

The True Story of a Bi-lateral Total Hip
Replacement Patient
A Serious, Technical and Sometimes Humorous
View on What You Can Expect and Might
Encounter Before, During, and After Hip
Replacement Surgery
Possibilities of a New Hip, or 2, and a New Life!

## JERRY RIEMER

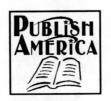

PublishAmerica
Baltimore

First printing

PublishAmerica has allowed this work to remain exactly as the author intended, verbatim, without editorial input.

ISBN: 1-60441-235-6
PUBLISHED BY PUBLISHAMERICA, LLLP
www.publishamerica.com
Baltimore

Printed in the United States of America

# TABLE OF CONTENTS

VOLUME II
HIP REPLACEMENT #2

I am dedicating this book and all its contents of hope and sincerity to the remembrance of my mother and father. My mother died of ovarian cancer several years ago at a relatively young age. She lost the fight for her life that makes any pain I have ever felt, pale in comparison. She was a very tough woman and the thought of her toughness and knowing her and God were there for me, helped me mentally through some bad times along my road leading up to and convalescing after my first hip replacement surgery. I thank God and my mother most every day for helping me.

My father passed away a few years after my mother. He died of cancer as well; Adenoe Carcinoma, a cancer that encompasses and surrounds every major organ in your body. Unlike my mom's fight, which lasted over a 5 year period, my father was taken away in less than 1 year.

I can tell you from experience it was hard being 38 years old and not having either of my parents around. It is a very sad feeling to have and I thank God my in-laws are still around, I love them as my mom & dad. They are two of the nicest people I've ever met. I often tell my wife and her siblings how lucky they (we) are to still have them around. They are in their 70's and we hope they are around forever.

My second dedication is to the Children's Hospital of Wisconsin and to the families that live out some bad times there. I feel the biggest tragedy in anyone's life as a parent is having something bad happen to their children. It is against the natural order of things to bury a child and I feel that it should never happen, but unfortunately it sometimes does. There was a story I saw on TV once, about a family that was blessed with a lovely young daughter. For a while she was fine, everything seemed to be normal. At the age of five, she was diagnosed with a disease that attacked her heart and lungs. The family went through hell, until finally God took the little girl to be with him. I cried through the entire story and am shook up while writing this even now. God works in mysterious ways and has a reason for everything he does. I am at a loss of understanding as to why things like that have to happen. To this family and other families like them, I hope their prayers are answered as my prayers concerning my hip were answered. Thank you Lord! I am not a Bible thumper, but I do believe God is up there, somewhere, and I draw strength from Him whenever I need to.

I would like to start by saying I am just an average guy. I am not a doctor, nor am I an expert on hip replacements or any medical procedures whatsoever. I am, however, a man that has had his life changed for the better due to the miracle of modern day medicine. I have benefited from two total hip replacements. I have lived through the trials and tribulations of dealing with chronic pain, a pain that was so intense at times it was changing who I was, how I felt and what I was becoming.

I am going to go through the stages or periods in my life that eventually led me to decide to have hip replacement surgery. I am going to show whoever reads my story, that it could in fact very well be their story too.

I am going to dedicate a portion of this book to the people whom have had this type of surgery done. I am doing this to show that they are the same type of people that have lived in agony like me until they could not handle the pain any longer.

I will also try to explain, with the help of documented research articles and my experience: exactly what the procedure entails, the possible ups and downs of the surgery, the possibility of complications or side effects, as well as the hope of a successful surgery and better quality of life because of it.

The purpose of this book is in no way intended to replace or act as a sole guide for rehabilitation, nor should it serve as guidelines by which a person should decide to have this surgery done. I have written in this book combining the experiences I've had and the research I've done in order to give people an idea of the process you go through in determining when the hip replacement should finally be done. I will go through my rehabilitation exercises as well as the other optional exercises on the road to recovery.

The absolute bottom line of anything you should decide to do in terms of surgery should be discussed with your family and a competent, well recommended surgeon. This is how you will build a structured plan by which you can change your life.

I not only speak from the experience of going through two total hip replacements, one on each side, but I have done a good amount of research as well. The contents in the rehabilitation/ technical chapter is a synopsis of what the majority of establishments in the medical field have determined to be the best overall rehabilitation venue for a rapid and complete recovery. Once again, if you are contemplating having any type of surgery done in this capacity, please seek out professional advice from a reputable physician/specialist. That way, together, you can figure out what would be the best way to treat your particular problem.

I feel that people need to hear my story because I think almost everyone knows somebody that walks with a limp, possibly due to a bad hip, or knows somebody that seems constantly agitated and/or edgy because of the pain in their hip. These people could be at their mental and physical breaking point because of hip pain, like I was. I will try to help these people understand that there is a procedure I call a modern day miracle, the total hip replacement. I have experienced it twice and I am proof that it can change their quality of life for the better.

If I only reach one person with this book and change their life for the better, then this book will have served its purpose. Nobody needs to live in pain.

Sincerely,
Jerry Reimer JR.

# VOLUME I
# HIP REPLACEMENT
# #1

# CHAPTER ONE:
## Growing Pains

I am going to start by saying my childhood was pretty normal. As long as I can remember I was always involved in some kind of sport. There were times when my dad would have me kicking a football in the house, when I was 4 years old or so, only to have the kicks go the wrong way and break a lamp or something. Boy, we sure caught heck from my mom when that happened. Those are memories I will always cherish. I recall in our house in the 60's, the Green Bay Packers with Vince Lombardi as coach were a very popular item on Sundays during the football season. Growing up, my brother and I would play football in the backyard. I was a bit older and a lot bigger than he was. In fact, with the way I pummeled him into the bushes next door, he should be the one with hip problems, not me. I would sing the opening kickoff song and proceed to pursue him after I booted it; most of the time I caught him, much to his dismay. I believe it made my brother tougher because of it, but of course I was the only one who could treat him like that. Let's just say I was doing it for "his own good". (Yeah, right!)

Other than the few bumps and bruises of a young child's life, I did not show any signs of abnormal hips or hip problems as the case would be later on.

God fortunately blessed me with decent athletic ability. As I got older into my 6, 7 and 8th grade years I developed into a pretty good athlete. I remember one of the highlights of my career as a young basketball player for St. Sebastians in Milwaukee was receiving the honor of All-Tournament in the Arch Diocesan Catholic Grade School Tournament. Presenting the trophies was none other than Rick Majeris. At that time he was an assistant coach at Marquette University. He then became the head coach of the Milwaukee Bucks, and is now the coach at Utah University.

I was also a pretty good football player, aspiring to play college football some day. Instead I got married to a lovely girl whom is now my wife of 26 years. Ask anyone who knows me; that in itself is quite an accomplishment…for her anyway!

All through High School I never showed signs of hip problems or any abnormalities health wise. I was heavy into lifting weights and still am today. Working out is something I love to do and hopefully I can still do in the years to come. Later on in life, I thought that lifting weights was part of the reason for my hip discomfort. This was the furthest from the truth, as I will get into later in this book.

Summing up my life through High School, I was pretty normal health wise. Mentally might be a different story, depending on who you ask! Athletically and physically, I was in pretty good shape, showing absolutely no signs of hip dysfunction or abnormalities, and no signs of arthritis…yet.

The bad news was yet to surface. Yes, unfortunately, the story gets worse, before eventually it gets better.

Stay with me…

# CHAPTER TWO:
## Career Choice/Turning Point

My father had always been a Printer/Lithographer his whole life. Thus, when I was 18, I had a wife, a new baby girl named Nichole Marie, and responsibilities that I needed to pay for. Naturally, my dad suggested I pursue a career that was in the trades, one that had provided his family with an honest, decent living...printing. With the help of a very dear friend of my fathers, I got my first job in the printing trade in 1980. I would like to take this opportunity to say that printing has been very, very good to me. I am a hard worker and 26+ years later I am running an 8-color press at a very nice shop called Burton & Mayer Printers and Lithographers in Menomonee Falls, WI. I have been there for 17 years and enjoy going to work.

The first 10 years of my printing career were very physical. I had the normal aches and pains that everyone else did. But still, up until 30 years of age, I showed no signs of hip problems or hip abnormalities. I was still working out with weights and entertained the thought of someday competing in an amateur body building contest. It was about this time I started to show signs of left hip discomfort. The pain would throb for a bit then subside. The amount of time spent on my feet would affect how much my hip would hurt. If I was working 12-hour shifts, it hurt a lot, but when I would sit down the pain would go away, so I thought nothing of it.

I continued working out and was actually gearing up for a body building competition at the Wisconsin State Fair in 1987. I remember looking pretty buff approaching 2 months before contest time.

This is when I had my first major setback. While playing basketball of all things, I attempted to throw a full court pass and felt a pop in my left bicep muscle. What felt like my arm was coming apart was actually my bicep tendon rupturing and tearing completely from my bone. While waiting for a diagnosis at the ER at West Allis Memorial Hospital, I can remember the pain was very bad. What was worse, was not knowing what was wrong. The attending physician at the ER wanted an orthopedic surgeon to have a look at it also. This was the first opportunity I had to meet the doctor that would eventually be the man that would change my life. The two doctors stood in front of me and discussed out loud that something was missing in my left arm, saying to each other, "It's not there, is it?" Of course, I immediately said, "What exactly isn't there?" The good doctors both said simultaneously, "Your left bicep tendon is not there, it's torn from your elbow!" I then asked them to explain what that meant and followed that up with when could I continue to train for my contest. Doctor James Wood informed me the rehabilitation would have to wait until after the surgery was done! A surgery was needed to reattach the tendon to the bone. He also added that time was of the essence because after 24 hours or so after the injury, the tendon would start to scar to wherever it ended up after it snapped, and that once that happened; it could no longer be repaired.

Wow! That was a shocker! Needless to say, with not many options, I opted to have the surgery the next day. The major point is it established a trust thing with Doc Wood. I felt he was looking out for my best interest, which he was. I felt comfortable with the way he handled the situation, and to this day have a great amount of respect and admiration for what he does and who he is. The surgery went well, as did the rehabilitation afterward. The contest I was training for went on without me, but in what seemed to be not time at all, I was back in the gym training again. I have some restrictions in reference to my arm, more in the way the bicep looks than anything else. None the less, I was back on track, thanks to Doc Wood and a good attitude. I feel most everything in life good or bad that you deal with, have better outcomes when you approach each situation with the best attitude possible.

As time moved on, my left hip joint was gradually getting worse. The hip was not to the point where it hurt all the time yet, but it was literally getting to be a pain in the butt. A couple of years passed, this was when I decided that my walking was no longer normal. The pain was almost all the time now; chronic you might say. My disposition was being affected as well. Little things that did not matter much seemed like big deals. I was angry at the fact that my hip hurt like it did. I was an angry old man at the age of 27. I decided it was time to have my situation diagnosed. I decided to contact an orthopedic surgeon to evaluate my hip. A surgeon I felt comfortable with, a doctor I had dealt with and had respect for. Fortunately, I had that doctor in mind, and set up an appointment to see Doctor Wood...

...this time for my hip.

# CHAPTER THREE:
## Hip Diagnosis/Prognosis

I knew it was time to see Doctor Wood. People kept asking me if I hurt myself because of the way I was limping around. I did not feel like working out anymore because of the pain affecting me, not only physically, but mentally as well. My attitude at home was getting to the point where it was affecting my relationship with my wife and kids. Everything seemed to unnerve me. I'm sure if you ask the people that really know me, they might say that is the way I am all the time, but all kidding aside, things were getting worse.

I saw Doctor Wood one morning in the fall of 1990. We had some pleasant conversation and then we got down to business. I remember the first thing he said was, "You're too young to have a hip in this kind of shape." At this point, he did not know why it was so bad. He took some x-rays to find out. He thought maybe it was Rheumatoid arthritis, oseoarthritis, or lyme disease. Lyme disease was a possibility because I was and am a taxidermist and there is always a risk in dealing with deer that have tics that could carry the disease.

As I was waiting for the Doctor to return with the x-rays, all I could think about was why I was having to deal with this hip problem; on one hand feeling pretty fortunate that I only had to deal with a problem that could be corrected, and not a life threatening illness such as cancer or diabetes, but on the other hand agreeing with the good doctor... "Why me" at 30 years old dealing with 90 year old hips?

The Doctor returned with the x-rays and that pretty much showed what the problem was. A close look at the ball and socket joints of my hip revealed the cartilage in both joints was very close to being nonexistent. The question was why. The Doctor proceeded to show me why. It appears that from birth, something was genetically wrong with my hip joints. There seems to be burrs on the ball of the joints, which caused the cartilage to be worn away.

As the Doctor and I talked, the nurse drew blood to test and see if I had another form of arthritis. We found out later there was not, which was good, but I still had a serious problem I had to deal with. My left hip was considerably worse than the right hip. Both were causing me discomfort and pain. The Doctor explained to me there were several options that I had:

The first option I had was to treat the pain with anti-inflammatory drugs. These drugs are designed to keep the joint and area around the joint from swelling which causes the pain. The drug I used was Voltarin. He explained to me that it can cause stomach discomfort, and that the drug works for some people, but also, that it is not a cure all to end all. I got the impression it was designed to mask a more serious problem, or to postpone the inevitable, which is a viable option. (At least for a while)

The second option was to fuse the joint to stabilize it. This is designed to immobilize the joint, the range of motion being almost nothing. Since there would be no movement in the joint, there would be no pain, but the quality of life would be limited in that you could not do much in the realm of sports or other strenuous activities involving your legs. Even though this was an option, it was not an option I wanted to pursue. I was only 30 years old and the thought of being restricted to certain movements did not interest me.

The third and final option was a total hip replacement. Cut the old one out and put a new, man made one in. There would be certain limitations with this one as well of course, but they were fewer than fusing the joint. The pain would be gone. Also, in the last few years up until my diagnosis, modern medicine had come a long way with hip replacements and the Doctor added that they will be even better in future.

Doctor Wood at this visit almost refused to even think about performing a fusion or hip replacement. He expressed concern that I was too young to have something like that done. He also said, "Why not try the oral anti-inflammatory drug first, maybe that would work for a while." He set me up with a prescription of Voltarin and said that my condition will only get worse and eventually lead to other options for a better quality of life. One of the biggest reasons for Doc Wood's advice to hold off on a replacement, was that the replacements at that time were only guaranteed for 10-15 years. That would mean I would have to, in all probabilities, have to go in for another replacement for the same hip at a later date. Not something I wanted to even think about.

# CHAPTER FOUR:
## The Next Few Years

I was 30 years old and pretty much dealing with the hand I was dealt. I had degenerating hip joints, and was trying to combat the pain with anti-inflammatory drugs. I would just grit my teeth when the pain got too bad. I was still training for the body building contest that I always wanted to compete in. I was also in the process of building a house and was working a lot of hours at my job as a lithographer. My left hip joint was getting really bad. My movements at the gym had to be really strict and well planned out as not to hurt myself more. Every movement lower body wise was painful, but I stayed focused and somehow managed to work through the pain. Looking back on it now, I don't know how I did it.

Along my journey to compete in the contest, I met and became friends with a very intelligent young man that worked as a physical therapist at the health club I belonged to. We became friends as I saw and talked to him almost every day. I eventually began calling him Professor Jon because of his uncanny ability to boggle people's minds with technical terminology about the body. He would give a scientific explanation when telling us how muscles worked and discuss the molecular breakdown of muscles and supplements and on and on, you get the picture. He was happiest when he was helping someone, health or otherwise. A wise man well beyond his years, he said something to me that I will never forget. He said, "Success is not measured by what you achieve, but rather by what you overcome." I often think of him to this day. He was and still is my friend to this day.

I had a chance to train with some Milwaukee Admirals in the weeks before my contest. I found out first hand just how intense a professional athlete has to train to prepare for a year of competition in their sport. I would not have believed it unless I actually experienced it myself, which I did. The most grueling of exercises that I will always remember and despise was the medicine ball sit ups. Jon would stand up about 5 feet from the incline sit up bench. At the steepest incline I would begin by sitting up and prepare to catch a medicine ball he would throw to me. I would catch the ball and throw it back while going down to do another repetition. Jon would move from left to right and back while continuing to throw the ball. After one set, I swear I could have had a car drive over my stomach it felt so hard and sometimes I wanted to throw up.

My hip pain was still very prevalent and persistent but with the workouts and anticipation of my contest I was able to put it in the back of my mind somehow. I was in the best shape of my life. I was 32 years old and was going into a bodybuilding competition. Competing against 20 year olds, etc…

The competition came and went. I remember directly after I placed third, out of twenty guys, how it felt kind of bittersweet. I was overjoyed with the feeling of accomplishment from all the work I put into the contest, but also a bit of sadness knowing how

I might never be in this kind of shape again because of my hip. There was a point that day where my emotions got the best of me. My trainer Jon put me over the edge when he gave my daughter something to give me later on that evening. It was a trophy with the saying I mentioned before. He knew the hip pain I dealt with while I trained. I feel in my heart he respected me because I worked through the pain and somehow blocked it out.

The house we had built was just about ready for us to move into by now. The work we had ahead of us was extensive; landscaping, painting, staining and general new house stuff. Lots of work to be done, so little time. Needless to say with our relocation and the work we had to do, my workouts became less and less of a priority, which I knew would be the case. The new house consumed most of our time. The kids were growing up fast and all of them were in extra-curricular activities such as sports, which even lessened my working out. Later in the years, I wasn't working out at all. This was saddening to me as I eventually got out of shape. Along with being out of shape, my hip was getting really bad. I was in such pain that I was trying to alleviate the pain by taking way too much Ibuprofen. So much, that I was taking them like candy. That was not good and that affected me as I will get into later.

I had a more important situation I had to deal with. My mother whom I adored and was one of my best friends was diagnosed with cancer. She was gearing up for the fight of her life. This fight lasted five years or so and she eventually lost the battle as she passed away. Valerie was one tough woman. I thought to myself with the things that woman had to go through, three major surgeries and a whole lot of pain, my hip pain was minuscule by comparison. I thought to myself I was being a baby about the pain, just take some more pills and tough it out. That was the worst thing I could have done.

In the next year or so, I had myself so medicated with pain pills that it affected my equilibrium. I was dizzy at work, I was irritated and restless, I couldn't sleep, etc. I didn't know at the time that it was the over medicating causing this, I thought the worst because of my mom's situation: I thought I had brain cancer. I was convinced I had something seriously wrong with my head. I always think the worst, it's just the way I am. I went to the clinic and they put me through all the blood tests and everything else. After a month or so they finally figured it was all due to me over medicating myself.

This was about enough to get me into the doctor for discussing the other options. Inevitably, a total hip replacement was probably going to be a reality.

# CHAPTER FIVE:
## Surgery Time Has Come

My mother's death was now a few years passed. Today, like most everyday, I think of her. I can still see her standing at the top of the stairs outside of our house on 58th and Vliet Street waiting for me to come home from grade school. I will be drawing from her strength to get through the hard times awaiting me in the future.

Now that my hip pain had just about taken over my whole persona, I realized it was time to explore my other options concerning my hip.

Again, enter Doctor Wood. I made an appointment and later that week I met with him apprehensively. I knew what he was going to say and I guess I really didn't want to hear it. He always left decisions up to me, so he presented options. He would help me with explanations and leave the bottom line up to me and my family.

He took x-rays again to see how much my hip had degenerated. He recorded a range of motion on both hips. There was almost no range of motion on my left hip. It was time to do some thinking about it. Even though I was the youngest patient Doctor Wood had performed a hip replacement on (at age 35), he agreed my quality of life could be vastly improved as a result of a successful surgery. He does not perform a surgery like this unless both he and the patient agree this is the way to go. Both Doctor Wood and myself agreed that my quality of life had degenerated and suffered because of my bad hip. It was time to do the surgery. He then explained somewhat of how the surgery goes and what to expect, good and bad. Later in the book I will dedicate an entire chapter to the technical side of the surgery. There was one thing I needed to do health wise before he would operate. I had a bad hernia, which Doctor Wood said I needed repaired before he could operate. This surgery through no fault of a doctor turned out to be a very bad experience, which I will get into in a later chapter. An experience that later impeded my recovery form my hip replacement.

There was a mental block I needed to overcome before we set a date for the hip replacement, I was truthfully scared to think of someone sawing my hip out, the one God gave me, to have a man made hip pounded into place. Part of my fear came from stories I had heard through the grapevine so to speak. One story in particular kept me from pursuing the surgery earlier. Here's the story…

I was having some cement work done at my house about a year earlier and at the time I was limping pretty badly. Very noticeable, so much that one of the workers asked why I limped so badly. I told him about my degenerating hip situation and that I was considering a hip replacement eventually. He then proceeded to tell me a horror story about his father. It appeared his father had gone for a hip replacement a few years before, when he was 70 years old. After the surgery, an infection set in his hip. The infection was so bad, the new hip had to be taken out until the infection healed. Then, after the infection cleaned up, the new hip would have to be reinstalled. A year later, he was still recovering. Not something I wanted to hear. It scared me so much I postponed the surgery as long as I could. It is a scary thing to think as a provider for a family you could possibly be out of commission somewhere up to a year — worst case scenario, but possible none the less. As I found out he has recovered quite well and now, at the age of 75, leads a fairly normal life. His age had absolutely nothing to do with the infection. It's just a possibility for this type of surgery. There are some negative possibilities connected with a hip replacement surgery. Infection, blood clots, and the possibility of dislocation or the parts the doctor installed could possibly break. The whole surgery, rehabilitation and most everything related to the surgery will be discussed in the next Chapter. Stay with me, It gets interesting.

# CHAPTER SIX:
## What You Should Know—
## Technical/Medical—
## About a Hip Replacement

This chapter is a bit longer than the other Chapters. There is a reason for this. I wanted to make sure I covered most everything of what to expect when undergoing a total hip replacement technically, medically, mentally, and physically; from start to finish.

The most important thing I need to stress to whoever reads this chapter is its contents are in no way intended to be medical advice. Contact and confide in your physician for medical advice.

The contents of this chapter were put together from my experience of undergoing two total hip replacements. The exercises I went through in rehabilitation and a lot of research. A good source of help in research was Virtual Hospital's Iowa Health Book.

In this hip replacement introduction I will be covering some of the causes, when to have it done, and the description of the hip replacement itself. I will also delve into what to do and expect the day of the surgery, preparing for the pre-op visit, what things you might encounter after surgery, what type of exercises to do in rehab, and how to approach and handle everyday activities. There are a number of do's and don'ts at home following surgery. You'll need to know these and be concerned with them — I hope that after you read this chapter you can go into your doctor with a general and somewhat informed view of what you are in store for. With this information you should be better prepared for the surgery.

In general Osteo & Rheumatoid Arthritis are two of the biggest causes of pain that leads to total hip replacements. Both types of arthritis cause deterioration of the joint cartilage. Treatment usually starts with, as in my case, some type of anti-inflammatory drug and or the use of a cane to take the pressure off of the inflamed joint. The exhaustion of such drugs with no further relief ultimately leads to fusion of the joint of total prostheses... a new hip. Total hip replacement is a surgical procedure to replace the old worn hip. The prosthesis consists of two components or parts. The first component is the hip socket, medical name acetabulurm, a cup shaped bone in the pelvis. The second component is the head or the ball of the thigh bone which is the femur. The surgical procedure entails removing the two parts of the hip joint and replacing them with smooth artificial parts. There are no ligaments or tendons to hold the components together. This fact is why you have to be careful not to overdo anything for the immediate time up to six weeks or so after the surgery. The artificial ball and stem are made up of strong metals, stainless steel, ceramics, or titanium. The goal of the Medical Society is to use a substance that will last a lifetime. It is very important that hip replacement patients be careful to avoid positions which might dislocate the hip components. In the early years of hip replacements, the components were affixed with a bone cement called methyl methacylate. The use of this bone cement was popular until pressure fitting the components was developed. Usually the doctor chooses this with younger patients, because of the longevity of such a procedure. These pictures are representations of a good hip and an arthritic bad hip. Notice the gap between the ball and socket joints of both the good and bad hip:

## THE GOOD HIP

The Good Hip

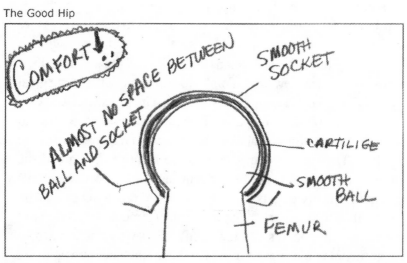

## THE BAD ARTHRITIC HIP

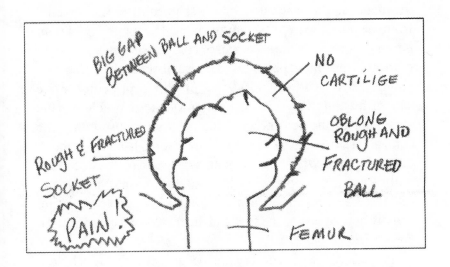

Total hip replacement is definitely major surgery and should be approached as such. The patient needs to know that with all major surgeries there are major risks. With this type of surgery, the risks include possible dislocation, infection, and loosening and breaking of components. Along with these are general medical complications that are possible such as blood clots in leg veins, (you will be required to wear nylons for a few days after surgery), pneumonia from lying around or anesthetic complications. A positive mental attitude is necessary before you enter surgery. Convincing yourself your life is going to change for the better because of the surgery is essential for a quick recovery. Trust me, it is not all hearts and flowers. The first few days directly after surgery I call HELL week!

In 90-95% of patients, a total hip replacement will provide relief from the pain that had been inhibiting you from normal everyday living. It will allow you to get back to work with a normal gate (walking normal); only under *your* physician's instructions. Most patients with a stiff hip joint will enjoy relief from the pain and improved movement. The longevity of your new hip varies with the activeness of the patient, and the weight of the patient. Obese people are not usually operated on as with young active patients. 90-95% of hip replacements are successful up to 10 years. The major long term problem is the loosening of the prostheses. This occurs because either the cement loses its adhesion, or the bone resorbs from the cement. 25% of all hips will show upon an x-ray looking loose. 5-10% will be painful. Loose hips can usually, but not always, be replaced. The results of a second total hip replacement are usually not as good as the first and the results of a complication are worse.

Preparing for your surgery must begin several weeks before your surgery. Good physical health is a *must* to endure the rigors of your surgery. A blood transfusion is often necessary after your hip surgery. I had to donate several pints of my blood prior to my surgery, so if I needed blood it would be my blood that I would get. This is called autologue blood donation. The first donation must be given within 42 days of the surgery and the last, no less than 7 days before surgery. I remember my doctor put me on some iron pills because they only accept your blood if you are healthy, without a cold or flu or infection because you could get this same illness when you recure your blood at the time of surgery. Your physician may order blood tests and a urinalysis two weeks before surgery as to insure no urinary tract infection is present. No infected teeth, or Gum Disease present, this infection could go to your hip, a bad situation. Also, as in my case, I needed to have my hernia repaired and healed before I could have my hip done. Your surgeon may ask you to see your family doctor to make sure you are in good enough health to endure the rigors of hip replacement surgery. When preparing for surgery you should think about the recovery period after surgery. Take it from me, you will not feel like your energy level is up to snuff. If help at home is not possible, you might want to make arrangements to stay a while in an extended care facility. I had a social worker that helped me figure everything out. That was nice. I also had a loving caring family prepared to help me in any and all ways possible.

I remember I had to make a pre-op visit to the hospital to go over some of the things to expect from my surgery before going home. I remember I watched a short film about the surgery. Also some detailed things gone over such as: following a regular diet on the day before the surgery, do not eat or drink after midnight, and a shower or bath should be taken the morning before surgery They gave me an antiseptic soap to use. The special soap contains iodine and reduces the risk of infection. We went over deep breathing exercises to minimize the risk of pneumonia or lung complications after surgery. As I mentioned before to reduce the risk of blood clots you will be required to wear elastic support stockings I call them (the medical name for them is TEDS). They aid in circulation because normal leg circulation occurs while walking, you will need something to take the place of that during the first few days of surgery. After my second hip replacement I had to inject myself at home with a blood thinner called Cumadin. There is an oral blood thinner you can take, but Cumadin is better. I had to check with my insurance company to see if they would cover the Cumadin. They did, so that is what I used.

Your surgeon may schedule an appointment with the anesthesiologist that will be handling your surgery to talk over possible medications on the day of your surgery. The pain control drugs will be administered directly into an IV the first few days after the surgery. I had a morphine drip which I could press as much as I wanted, but actually only dispersed a small amount of drugs every ten minutes no matter how much I pressed. The days following that period the nursing staff administers oral pain medication or if necessary, shots. Not alcohol, but rather needles. A very important reminder is to take the pain medication every so often as not to chase the pain. If you wait too long between doses, you may be sorry.

As with any major surgery, I suppose depending on your hospital policy of course, the day of surgery your family can accompany you on the elevator and then they have to wait in the waiting room. The doctor will come out after surgery and let them know how things went. The actual surgery may take 2-4 hours. After the surgery you will be taken to the recovery room for a period of close observation usually 1-3 hours. Your blood pressure, pulse and temperature will be checked frequently. The circulation and feeling sensation in your legs and feet will be monitored closely. It is very important to let your nurse know of numbness, tingling, or pain in your legs or feet. When you awaken and your condition is deemed stable, you will be taken to your room. Here are a few things you may encounter after surgery: You will have a large Band-Aid or dressing which will be changed 2-4 days after surgery. I know my dressing was totally saturated the day after and they did not change it, they just put another one over it. I did not have a hemovac suction container with tubes that led to my wound. I'm not sure why. You may have a hemovac, as it enables the nursing staff to monitor the amount of fluid that secretes from the wound and they measure and record the results. If you have a hemovac it's usually removed by a doctor 2 or 3 days after surgery.

As I mentioned before, an IV is started prior to surgery and will continue until you are taking proper amounts of liquid orally. Antibiotics and pain medications will be administered through the IV for as long as necessary to reduce the risk of infection. A catheter may be administered to allow the patient a passage way for urine. Preventing blood clots is very important, along with your stockings (TEDS) there may be an additional stocking applied which is hooked up to a machine which aids in circulation and the prevention of clots. You will also be given medication and exercise instructions to reduce the possibility of clots. You may feel nauseous and vomit after the operation due to the anesthesia; anti-nausea medication may be given to minimize those symptoms. As you can see, the nursing staff and your physician have just about anything at their disposal to eliminate any type of discomfort you might have, so don't hesitate to ask or tell them of things you are feeling and are concerned about. I did. Your diet will be allowed to progress as your condition gets better or permits. Coughing and breathing deep are important to help prevent lung complications such as congestion or pneumonia. Some patients, such as myself, experience back pain or discomfort after the surgery. Most of this is caused by the pain in the hip area or prolonged lack of mobility after surgery. Periodically changing positions will help to relieve the discomfort and prevent skin breakdown, which can lead to bed sores. The head of your hospital bed should not be elevated. The possibility of dislocation is actually a concern up to 6 to 8 weeks after surgery. Precautions need to be followed for this not to happen. One is not to cross your legs and not allow this to happen. The use of 2-3 pillows between your legs should do it. It feels good as well in the fetal position. Do not over bend, 90 degrees is way too far forward. The use of a high rise toilet seat took some getting used to, but you will experience that for yourself. Also the use of a grabber, a mechanical pair of fingers you will use to put on your socks, and generally use to get dressed, this takes some getting used to.

The first day after surgery you will actually begin therapy, physical by nature, but believe me, mental therapy may be needed later. You will first sit in a reclining chair, then you will gradually begin to take steps, walk, and then learn to go up and down stairs with the use of a walker or crutches. Initial rehabilitation takes 5-7 days. Some discomfort might be felt during the time in muscles that were cut during surgery, but my hip pain was miraculously gone.

Following surgery you will work with a physical therapist to progress to the point of being able to walk on your own with the aid of a walker, go up and down stairs, get in and out of bed and do exercises to improve your range of motion and strengthen your muscles surrounding your hip. A home exercise program will be mapped out with your therapist as well. Walking is not a substitute for exercise—take it from me—attack those exercises diligently and with purpose and focus, for these exercises will be the avenue for you to get back to a normal life. Remember the differences between good pain and bad pain. If needed, reduce your intensity. If a bad pain persists, call your physician. If dislocation occurs my doctor said he'd be able to hear my screams from his office, I live 20 miles away. So don't do anything stupid. I heard a story about a woman whom had the surgery and shortly after had to paint her toenails, needless to say, I don't think she did that after they redid her hip!!! Be smart, use your head, and listen to what your body tells you.

There is a variety of exercises that you will be asked to perform during your rehabilitation period and it's good to continue them for the rest of your life to maintain the strength and range of motion of your hip.

When you are discharged to go home, you will have a certain degree of independence in walking with crutches and climbing and descending stairs and general getting around. You are not, by any means, back to normal. You will probably need assistance around the house for a while so asking people to help you with certain things at first is part of the rehabilitating process. This part I had a hard time with. I thought I did not need anybody—I was wrong. *Let them help!* You will continue to take medication as prescribed by your doctor. Some may include blood clot prevention. Pain control medicine will also be prescribed. Remember when taking this type of medication it is necessary to be done as indicated—nothing more, but take it when it says to, controlling the pain is a lot better than chasing it. You must continue to walk with crutches and a walker as directed by your doctor, therapist, or physician. Rehabilitation exercises will dictate just how well you get, and how fast!

Avoid sitting more than an hour at a time. Do not cross your legs. It's best to keep your legs 12-18 inches apart. Always sit in a chair with arms. The arms provide a leverage to push yourself up to a standing position. A high kitchen bar type stool works well in the kitchen. Avoid the cushy, low type chairs; they tend to force your body into a 90 degree angle to get out of them which is BAD. Use your raised toilet seat, it is very satisfying, a day you'll look forward to, I promise. Remember, I speak throughout this book in the first person; I've been through it all, twice 11 years apart, both sides. You must not for the first 8 weeks following surgery bend over to pick up anything. Use your long handled grabber and a pair of slip on shoes for this period. Using your grabbers to put socks on, later in your rehabilitation, is quite a chore. This is something that brings people to laugh, if they are watching you. Suggest to them, "Funny? Why don't you try it and then I can laugh!"

Driving is not recommended for up to 6 weeks after surgery. When getting into a car, back up to the seat of the car, sit and slide across the seat toward the middle of the car keeping your knees 17-18 inches apart. Unfortunately sexual intercourse will probably not be on your mind for awhile, but eventually it does cross it. Sexual activity can usually resume after 2 months following surgery. You can usually return to work within 3-6 months or as instructed by your doctor, depending upon what you do for a living.

Showers are out until staples are removed and do not sit in a bathtub until the doctor says okay. Your incision needs to be clean and dry, also be aware of how it appears to be healing. If swelling, increased pain, drainage or redness occurs around the incision or you contract a fever, report this immediately to your doctor. In 3 weeks, if all is well, staples are removed.

The prevention of infection is very important, both at distant areas like strep throat or pneumonia, and locally at the hip. Antibiotics should be administered right away as to not allow infection to lodge at the hip. Dental work needs special attention in case a bacterial infection occurs. You need to tell any doctor/dentist/or physician that does work on you in the future, that you have a prosthetic hip. This will dictate how they go about medicating you.

Most return appointments following surgery are around 6 weeks after discharge from the hospital. At this time, x-rays will be taken to see how the hip has taken to your body. Subsequent visits will be scheduled as needed to monitor your new hip.

**The next paragraph is very important. It is subjective and explains when to have a hip replacement.

The total hip replacement is an elective operation, it is not a matter of life or death, per say. But a successful operation can change an individual's life for the better, as it did mine. Before a total hip replacement, there are options that you will exhaust. The final decision to have an operation should not be made by your doctor, or friend, or relative, but rather by *you*, because it is you that must face the risks and possible complications. You and you alone must take a look at your quality of life when get to the point of considering the operation. Has the pain in the hip caused you to change who you are, what you do, and who you are becoming? As for myself, I was an angry old man at the age of 35.

With a final overview, remember your doctor, physical therapist, and nursing staff are working for you to help you get your life back with this new hip, your own modern day miracle. The real success of the entire operation however, depends greatly on you. How focused and deliberate your exercise and rehabilitation program is and how carefully you apply the principles of home care and self-limitation. Oh yeah, I left one thing out, probably the most important thing…

Ask God to walk with you through this. Along with him, your best friends are your doctor, your physical therapist, and your family members.

Sincerely,
Best of Luck and may God bless you as He has me!

# CHAPTER SEVEN:
## First Things First

I mentioned earlier that Doctor Wood, my orthopedic surgeon, said I had to have my hernia fixed and healed before he would perform the hip replacement. So, I met with my family doctor, and he recommended a doctor, that worked out of a Hartford clinic in Wisconsin, whom he knew that specialized in hernia repair. I will first say the bad experience I mentioned I had was in no way the fault of any doctor. On the contrary—the doctor whom performed the hernia repair was not only competent but to this day I feel served me well. I have nothing but good things to say about the surgery itself and how I was treated at the Hartford clinic. Outstanding and I mean it. Here is what happened. I came out of recovery from the surgery a bit sore. It is day surgery; hence you go home the same day. I left the hospital in the afternoon and a couple days later was recovering rather comfortably with minimal abdominal pain. My hip was giving me more problems because of my weakened stomach muscles. By the end of the week, I thought I was okay. In fact, the thought of having my hip replaced had kind of been put into the back of my mind. Boy was I wrong. Friday came around, I was off work and I remember waking up in the A.M. We had a water bed so sometimes it was a bit of a chore getting over the bumper on the side. This morning was difficult. I got on the bumper, sat on it and proceeded to hop off the side onto the floor. That's exactly what I did. I landed flat on the floor. I had tried to stand on my legs as I hopped onto the floor, but there was a pain in my back I had never felt before, an excruciating pain that put me flat on the floor. The kids were in school and my wife was at work. No one was around but my sweet heart of a dog that was upsetting because I could not play with her. All I could do was cry and lay there on the floor, for quite a while. I did not, at this point, know exactly what was going on. All I knew was that it hurt and hurt badly. My back was spasming from one side of my body back to the other side. I eventually could not take the pain any more and decided I best try and heave myself up and get downstairs to the main floor. I also thought if I could get up and walk it off like a good hit in football, I'd be alright. Boy was I wrong. It took me 1 hour to get down the hall and down 15 steps to the kitchen. When I finally got there I stood in one spot for the next hour and cried a puddle of tears, literally. The floor was wet with tears of pain. I managed to get through that, and when the spasms subsided somewhat, I made a call to Doctor Wood, my Orthopedic surgeon. He informed me I probably pinched my sciatic nerve, something that curses me to this day. He explained, in between my winces of pain that because of the last few years walking like an old man, coupled with weak abdominal muscles because of the hernia repair, my nerve had found a new place to rest; unfortunately, in a spot it could be easily pinched. He then prescribed muscle relaxer pills and pain medication that I had my wife pick up on her way home. At this point before I got off the phone I told the Doc that it was time to cut me open. I told him as long as we're going to do one hip why not just do them both at the same time! I told him I was sick of living in chronic pain, and to just cut me in half and put the new stuff in. I did not care about any possible downside of anything. I had had it. My hair was almost totally grey. I was a 90 year old man in a 35 year old man's body. I was at my point of no return. I told him I finally reached that point; I couldn't take it any longer. I was in agonizing pain, something I had never felt before and mostly because of my bad hip.

He calmed me down and proceeded to tell me never in a million years would he do both hips at the same time. He would not do both hips because it would be too hard to rehabilitate both at the same time. Your possibility of dislocation would increase greatly because you wouldn't have one good leg to rely on and that once I healed up from the hernia, and I would, that we would schedule the hip replacement, and only then, would he do it. I reluctantly agreed. I set the date 5 weeks from my bad day…Friday, March 20th, a day that I will always regard as Good Friday.

# CHAPTER EIGHT:
## Good Friday Is Finally Here!

During the course of the week prior to my surgery, I had some things I had to do to prepare. One of which you need to donate your own blood in case you need it after or during the surgery—better to use your own blood than someone else's. The weird thing about that is if they don't use it they throw it out. I don't' quite understand that, but that's why I'm not a doctor.

Yes. I was feeling some anxiety, and my sciatic nerve was still somewhat pinched—so you can picture how I was walking now. Very gingerly and looking not only like an old man, but a crippled old man! I kid you not.

Everything checked out and Friday had arrived. I was not to have any food after midnight the night before, (I call that bad Thursday and I don't think I slept too well that night).

We woke up the morning of the surgery and I remember feeling pretty good about what was about to happen. Good thoughts of ridding myself of a chronic hip pain that had plagued me most of the last 10 years of my life. My wife and I went about our normal routines of getting ourselves ready to shortly be on our way to the hospital.

She had something to eat while I wished I could eat something. There wasn't too much conversation between us. I know I was in and out of deep thought. She was just trying to keep things light. I remember thinking about my mom and what must have been going through her mind while she waited to go in for her surgeries for cancer. My surgery while being major, was nothing compared to someone facing their own mortality. The thought of that helped me stop feeling sorry for myself. I said my good-bye's to my kids and proceeded to be on our way to the hospital. I recall both wishing the trip to the hospital would be quick and long. One minute I wanted us to be there, the next minute I wanted to be 1000 miles away. Don't ask me what that was all about. Freud would have a field day with that.

Before I knew it, we were there at the hospital admittance desk. They all had smiles on their faces. I'm sure I did not!

My wife took care of the paper work while a nurse took me to the waiting room to get changed. My wife then met up with me, while then we both waited impatiently for me to be bedridden away.

The time went by very slowly it seemed. I'm not sure, but I think we only waited for less than one hour. I know it seemed like days to me. Too much time to think about stupid stuff like dying! I know it was absurd to think about that, but you know what they say about idle minds. Everything was running through my mind, mostly bad stuff. I couldn't help myself. It just kept snowballing until I think I farted and that for some stupid reason, made all of us laugh and lightened things up until I was on my way down the hallway. I was looking up at the ceiling and the lights going by and hoping one of the lights was my guardian angel looking over me to make sure I'd be all right.

We finally got to the operating room and they, on the count of three, transferred me to the table. The anesthesiologist administered the knock-out medication and I proceeded to count backwards 10, 9, 8… nighty-night bunny rabbit…

I don't recall how long I was actually under the knife, so to speak, but I do recall waking up in the recovery room. The first thing I remember is waking up a bit groggy to a voice of a nurse. She said to me, "How do you feel?" In a matter of seconds I felt a pain that sent me into a fit. It wasn't my hip; it was my cursed sciatic nerve. My back was so pained I almost passed out. The odd thing is, that even with the intense back pain; miraculously I could not feel any pain in my hip area. I can honestly remember explicitly that there was no pain at all in my hip. I could not believer it, as they sedated me with pain medication to relieve my back discomfort, I recall my eyes tearing up— realizing the possibility of my hip pain being gone. A miracle. In my mind I recall a conversation I had with my nurse in the recovery room. The pain medication was almost immediately effective. As I was calming down we had a real nice conversation. I thanked her for helping me and I remember I did not feel any pain after a few minutes. Once the pain medication was working, everything was great. No worries at all. I was in little Jerry, Jerry land and everything was okay…for now. I then went back to sleep. The worst was yet to come. I will now go into my 6 day diary of the recovery stay in the hospital. Some anecdotes are humorous, others are somewhat sad, and some will explain the pain I had to deal with, none of which was in my hip.

# CHAPTER NINE:
## Surgery Diary:
## From the Day After Surgery
## 'Til My Release Home

The first day I can remember I was hooked up to a morphine drip. An I.V. that had a button which I was able to push as many times as I wanted, but would only administer a small amount of pain medication once every 10 minutes, no matter how many times I pushed it. Believe it when I say pain and I have a love-hate relationship...I love to hate it. I am not a "baby," so to speak, but I am also not one who is too much of a man to admit I have pain and take something to alleviate the pain. I think I must have pushed that button a hundred million times...

For the first 24 hours immediately following the surgery, the staff was assigned to watch me and did just that. My temperature was monitored; my heart-rate, blood pressure and other vitals were regularly checked. I remember I had male nurse students aspiring someday to be doctors. They were very nice and watched me very well. I felt comfortable with them. I had a massive band-aid on the incision and remember them changing it once or twice. I was on the morphine drip, and I was not in any discomfort, except for the back pain. As I went over in a previous chapter, the sciatic nerve had to be physically moved in order to do the procedure. This did not help now, as I was already experiencing back pain before all this. For the most part, everything was going all right, at least as good as could be expected.

Doctor Wood visited me a couple times that first day. When I was coherent enough to talk to him I remember him sitting in the chair telling me everything went well, and that his arms were sore from pressure fitting the spike in my femur. He suggested that was a good thing because my bones were very hard and in good shape. He then told me that the hip joint itself was so deformed from being so sloppy that it was almost unrecognizable. It was definitely time to do the surgery and probably too long coming. So here is a suggestion to all whom are contemplating this surgery. You don't have to wait until your leg almost falls off. The bottom line for deciding if you should have this surgery lies within yourself. If your quality of life has digressed to the point of not being able to do normal everyday functions, it is time to get your life back, so to speak. Take it back by using the modern day medical technology we have at our convenience. You will be surprised. No, it's not an easy road. Yes, there are road blocks and speed bumps, detours and delays, but with the help of God, family and friends, you've got to believe you will get better and eventually your life will be normal again.

The second day was much of the same, everything as far as my vitals were being checked regularly. I still had the morphine button hooked up and I was using it. More for the back pain than anything else. I am truthfully going to say this again. I was experiencing absolutely no hip pain at all. I was scheduled to have a nurse and a therapist, show me how to properly use crutches. The therapist showed up in the afternoon and took me down to the practice floor, where there was a room with steps, etc… to practice with my crutches. The first sessions went well. I was up the second day, using my crutches. My back was still a sore spot, but I thought and was told that would probably go away. Later on you'll find out everyone was wrong. The Doc was weaning me off the morphine drip and was having me use oral pain pills (Vicadin) for discomfort. After all my second day recovery was successful. I must tell you I was not eating much, not because I was ill, but because I did not want to go to the bathroom in a bed pan. Don't ask me why, I just have something against bed pans. I don't like them! I remember one time visiting a friend of mine whom had had surgery on his knee. I was told I could bring him lunch to the hospital and I did. I brought him a submarine sandwich, and I had one also. Both he and I loved onions. I ended my visit and returned home. Later on that evening, I came out of the bathroom and unknowingly left the bathroom door open. Immediately my family complained of an awful smell…as if someone had died…I can only imagine the look on my buddy's nurse's face when she came for *HIS* bed pan!

This day was significant in the fact I was able to use my crutches and walk around the floor I was on. I was told that a few steps to the first nurse's station would be good progress. I remember feeling real well and I have a very competitive attitude. The few steps with the therapist weren't enough for me. I remember when she left; I waited a while and ventured out on my own, going up and down the floor, talking with people and having a good time. I felt good about everything that was going on. I thought the worst was over and all good things would be coming my way. Once again I was wrong, as I will get into later. For now, I was thanking God, my back pain was there but not intense, I was on the rehabilitation road and I was driving not Miss Daisy, but rather myself, but I was not prepared for the road block coming just ahead...

This day was one I would rather not talk about. To this day I get the shakes and a sick feeling in my stomach when I talk or even think about Hell Day.

Up until now I had a few visitors each day. Mostly close immediate family, my wife, a couple cousins, my dad and my wife's mom and dad. You really appreciate people who visit you when you're in a hospital. It can seem a cold and lonely place most of the time. A friendly face can really pick your spirits up. You don't ever forget, at least I don't, who took the time out of their schedule to go out of their way to come and spend a little time with me. I am greatly appreciative of all who came to see me. Even though I said not to come!

I will pick up Hell Day the evening before. About 9:00 p.m. My wife was just about to leave and I had told her I wasn't feeling the greatest and that I would like her to call me later to check on me. She left and I remember it was down hill after that. The lights were out and I wasn't interested in watching T.V. I read a lot, but this particular night I just chose to fall asleep, thinking about nothing, nothing at all. I'm not sure what followed was because of me coming off the morphine or what, but I was truly scared…

I remember waking up with my teeth chattering and feeling very cold and alone. If it weren't for the door being cracked and seeing a little light I think I would have done something like yell or scream or something.

When I woke up, I did not know who I was, where I was, or what I was doing there. The next 30 seconds or so I remember freaking out because my bed was soaking wet, I had my legs tangled in covers and was trying furiously to kick them off. Yes, kick them, I forgot I was rehabilitating a total hip replacement and a few more kicks let me know. I felt pain in my hip and back while trying to swing my body out of the bed, once

I felt that pain I came back to my senses. Seeing my walker and crutches drew me back into reality. My teeth were now chattering so loud and intense, that with every chatter, my back hurt more and more. I was now feeling like the scene in "Titanic" where all the people are out in the water freezing to death waiting to be rescued. Just what I was doing? I was freezing and now crying and standing on my walker next to the bed. I was trying to compose myself but could not. I proceeded to take small steps with my walker over to the window in my room. I shoved myself into the chair next to the window and sat there crying for the next few hours. It was 3:00 a.m. in the morning. I did not move from that chair, for the next 12 hours I was mentally drained and physically exhausted.

I proceeded to tell everyone that came into my room that day to abruptly leave—the therapist, the nurse, my family…even God.

I don't exactly know what happened to this day, but it was no fun. Later in the day I had two visitors at separate times. The first visitor was my Aunt Nancy. She is a lovely woman and a close friend and relative. She would take nothing less than me physically coming over to see her in the other part of the room. I explained in no uncertain terms I wanted nothing to do with visiting or anything else for that matter. Like I said she was stubborn and said she could wait for days and would if that's what it took. What could I do? I went over to her in my wheel chair and proceeded to visit unwillingly.

By the end of 10 minutes or so she had me laughing a bit and I was glad she came. She made me eat something before she would leave. I kissed her goodbye and wheeled myself back to the window. Boy, I really love that woman, she probably doesn't know how much, but I hope she reads this and realizes how much her visit meant to me.

I thought I was over that feeling of loneliness and emptiness...I was wrong. Soon after she left depression set in again and I was back staring at the window feeling sorry for myself.

Some time went by and the second of my two visitors showed up, my Uncle Bill. He is a man I respect greatly and could do nothing less than listen to him talk to me. He offered words of encouragement and told me that this wasn't the nephew he knew. The nephew he knew was a fighter and a winner, both of which I had lost sight of. He left, and I concentrated on getting my attitude back. It eventually came back and I felt a little better, but my back pain was very prevalent now. I insisted the Doctor come and see me and insisted that he x-ray my back again. Reluctantly he did, and seemed a bit perturbed with me. He said before the x-ray he could operate on my back, but did not want to. I did not at this point know what I wanted. I came back after x-ray and I got emotional again. I cried for a while and went to sleep. For now Hell Day was over, a 24 hour visit to Hell. A place that is not nice to live in, or visit for that matter.

Once again, I would like to thank my Uncle Bill and Aunt Nancy for keeping me from completely losing my mind that day.

I slept for quite a while after the worst day of my life. I woke up telling myself that I was going to be OK; that things were going to be better. My back didn't feel too bad, that was nice. I was taking less and less pain pills and took my last therapy session. They felt confident that I was able to manage the crutches and get around. Up until now, I had not gone to the bathroom. I refused to go in a bed pan. They would not let me leave the next day unless I had a bowel movement. I was getting nervous. I might end up going in a bed pan. I remember late in the evening my back pain was back, the x-rays came up negative. Everything was in place, nothing according to the x-rays was wrong, yet I was in a lot of pain. I remember crying and having the nurse come in. She hugged me and told me that maybe this is the way it was going to be. She said some people just don't get better. In fact, maybe I had to deal with it. I immediately stopped crying and feeling sorry for myself. I then told her no way was this how it was going to be. I would show her! She went away and I went to sleep with purpose. I was going to get through this back pain! I was going to be all right!

My attitude was back on track, the doc wanted me to stay an extra day to make sure mentally I was alright. I still had not gone to the bathroom yet! I knew what I had to do!

I summoned the nurse. I said I needed a suppository. She asked why. I said because I had not gone to the bathroom yet. She said she would be back to install it. I said, "No you won't." We went back and forth a few minutes and she finally gave in. I would administer the suppository myself.

Minutes later, nature called, I was there to answer. She was knocking on my door, and I needed to get seated quickly. Not an easy task for a hip replacement patient. You purchase a raised toilet seat so you don't sit down all the way and risk dislocation, so the seat was there, I had stared at it all week. I was now going to test drive it.

Minutes later, I was spelling relief and singing songs.

Tucked back into my bed, I anxiously awaited the nurse to tell her I had done my duty—but I wanted out of the hospital so bad I needed for her to believe that I went or they wouldn't let me leave…so I left her a present in the bathroom. The proof I needed to get out!

She came in with a grin on her face thinking I hadn't gone to the bathroom yet. I remember the look on her face when she came out of the bathroom. Sometimes pictures or a look is worth a thousand words. Her face said it all…I was going home!

Home is a very nice place to be and later on today I was going to be there. I was so excited. This chapter is very short because...

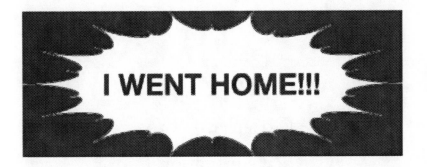

I WENT HOME!!!

I will add that the staff at the hospital was very friendly and very helpful the days I was there after my surgery. I felt very comfortable with the people and trusted them with my life.

I had reservations about actually going home. I knew that the rehabilitation was now going to be my job. I was going to get better only by how much I wanted to. I still had the back pain, but I will say other than overdoing the movement when my hip felt like it might dislocate, there was absolutely...

NO PAIN IN MY HIP!

I must have thanked the doctor a million times and God as well.

I was now on the road to recovery and hopefully a new life with my new hip! I was not out of the woods, but the clearing ahead was now visible. I was excited.

# CHAPTER TEN:
## Rehabilitation Is
## Exhilarating and Frustrating

While I was lying around the first few weeks I was able to think about a lot of things. I don't particularly like to watch a lot of TV; I would rather read or just think. I had an opportunity to do a lot of soul searching as well. I made a point to change some things I did not like about myself and vowed to get back in the contest shape I was in years earlier. It would not be easy. Even with my God given hips it wasn't easy. The thought of training that hard again with a prosthetic hip, I could almost not fathom. But it did not deter my hopes to be there again. Up on that stage with nothing but my posing trunks and my body—I willed it to be so.

I remember I started slowly at first. What else could I do? First I needed to get my muscles that were cut during the operation back functioning again. Getting the flexibility of the joint itself needed tending to as well.

I would lie on the floor and do leg lifts at first, then later would bring my knees up to my chest. (Look into the exercises for the hip in another part of this book). The doc knew I was active before and was anxious to get back training, but he had restrictions. There'd be no running, the jarring motion impact on the joint would not be good and no heavy squats with weights. I did not like to do either of these, so now I had an excuse. I could however bike, which I loved to do and work out within my limits, upper body wise, until my heart was content.

I started slowly mind you and was making good progress— it seemed 3 weeks into rehab, I was making very good progress. My flexion on the joint was about 85%. It also seemed that since I was walking more normal, my right hip felt a hundred times better as well. My back pain was finally subsiding and I was beginning to think the worst was over; Once again, I was wrong.

I can remember the first time I rode my bike. It was only to the corner and back, but the feeling of success that I had was incredible. Each day I would go a little further until one day I was feeling pretty good and I was about 2 miles away from home. I remember it was a beautiful spring day in April. I looked at one of the biggest hills in my area and thought I would try and tackle it. I headed towards it and started up it. Half way up I could feel my heart pumping vigorously. I probably should have quit right there, but I'm foolish so I continued up the steep incline. I couldn't believe I was doing this less than a month after a total hip replacement, but I was. Upon the completion of the hill, I had to stop to catch my breath. I was breathing very heavily and then emotion took over me. I got off my bike and started crying—tears of joy I think. Breathing heavy and crying don't go well, and a farmer near by came over to see if I was alright. I nodded, and uttered a few words to that effect. No, I was riding high. I conquered Norwegian Hill, and I could not wait to get back to the house to call everyone and tell them the good news.

A week went by and another major road block. I was not out of the woods, and maybe this was a sign I was over doing it a bit. I recall I was doing some side bends and had just woken up. Maybe I wasn't stretched out enough or I don't know what, but my old nemesis returned again. The back pain! I could not believe it, I thought I was over it. I was not. For the next 10 days I fought back from the pinched nerve that probably will plague me for life. I want to tell you again though it was not because of the hip surgery—it went back to the hernia repair.

It was time to get rid of the water bed. There was no stability with that bed. We needed to get a more firm mattress and did away with the water bed. That helped. Before long I was back on the rehab trail, getting better by leaps and bounds now; ridding myself of some un-needed body weight and working out more and more each day.

I was still not back to work yet—scheduled return was July 1st, a couple weeks away.

By now I was feeling good and looking good. I thought I had it made. Last visit with the doc was a couple days away and I was anxious to show him my shape.

I will remember the last visit for the rest of my life. I can recall my emotions like it was yesterday. While driving to the doctor's office, I was already getting emotional to the point of almost crying. As I pulled up to the office I composed myself, at least for now. I walked in the office and there were a lot of people there. I can remember the doctor was by the front desk and I lost it. I was weeping a bit and grabbed him and kissed him on the cheek thanking him and telling everyone because he gave me my life back. He changed my life, as if God had done a miracle that's how I felt.

The good doctor was a bit embarrassed, I'm sure, but I wanted everyone including him to know how grateful I was for what he had done for me. I say it was a miracle. I got what you would call a second chance. Believe me, I am going to make the most of it, you can too.

# CHAPTER ELEVEN:
## My Family Tells
## Their Story

This chapter is dedicated to my family. It is their opportunity to tell you how they perceived me before surgery and today. Here are their stories.

ASHLEY'S STORY:
(age 7-1/2)

Before my dad had his hip replacement, he would limp and complain about how much it hurt. After the surgery, the doctor's told him it would be awhile until he could ride a bike or workout, but a few days later, he was walking the hallways of the hospital. When he got home, he was a little grumpy. But after awhile, he seemed to be happy again and it's a lot nicer when he's happy.

## JEREMY'S STORY:
(age 12)

I remember my dad always being grumpy, never wanting to play. This was, of course, when I was younger and my father was having problems with his hip. At the time, I had no idea what was happening, but I soon found out that the man I called dad would be going under the knife. How was I to know that he would come out a whole different person? His attitude had changed completely. Now he is more active than I am. My father's hip replacement had not only changed his life, but everyone's lives around him.

## NIKI'S STORY:
(age 16)

In my eyes, my father has always been a person to look up to in the areas of personal dedication and achievement. Throughout my life, I have witnessed my father take on countless challenges and never once have I seen him quit. The range of these challenges includes every area of life; whether it be related to family, career, social, or physical activity, he has conquered them all. He has succeeded in all he has done, so I knew that the recovery from this surgery would not be his first failure.

The surgery was clearly necessary. No document or x-ray was needed for us to see that this was true. This conclusion was made simply by seeing his decline in physical activity and amount of pain that he was going through.

It was very hard to see my father struggle with something as simple as walking after the surgery. It was also very difficult to accept the fact that there was nothing I or anyone else could do to make his recovery go faster or to lessen his pain. I have always known my father to be a pretty up beat and motivated person, but there were periods of time after surgery where upbeat was not exactly the word for his mood. But in time, his motivation was back, and he was back to his normal fun loving, goofy self. He is now able to do things like lift weights and bike ride. You know, they say that after a hip replacement you have many physical limitations, but by looking at my Dad, you wouldn't be able to tell.

## MY WIFE LYNN'S STORY:

When I first met Jerry, he was somewhat of a super athlete. He was involved in many competitive sports in high school, such as football, basketball, and track. He also ran miles around his house to keep in shape. Jerry competed with such intensity and drive in everything he took on, he was very good and strong.

After high school was over, Jerry and I married. I thought maybe his activities would slow down, but I was wrong. He took up racket ball, biking, and continued with even more intensity in body building. He was extremely fit.

Life was pretty normal for us, we had three healthy, beautiful kids. Jerry and I were pretty involved with teaching them how to play baseball, basketball, etc…Jerry loved to run around with the kids and roughhouse; he was like a big kid himself.

I'm not exactly sure when it was, when Jerry started to get irritable after a lot of activity. I think it was shortly after Ashley, our youngest, was born, maybe '88 or '89. Jerry would get frustrated by this pain in his leg or back. Then the crabby years started. He became less involved with the kids, over time, and crabby to me.

Of course, like most men, Jerry didn't seek medical advice right away. I guess he thought whatever it was, he could beat it. He tried heat creams, hot baths, back pills, aspirin and anything else he could think of. He even gave up most of his recreational sports. But not weight lifting, he was determined to be in the Mr. Wisconsin Body Building Contest.

Jerry started limping, gradually at first, until about 1990. The limp was so bad, it hindered him, which was finally intolerable, so he went to see Dr. Wood. He was so young and walked like he was an old man. The Doctor said he needed a hip replacement, but suggested he held off as long as possible because he was so young and the artificial hips didn't last forever. What a horrible thing to hear for such and athlete, we were thinking maybe it was a bone spur, something easily corrected, and we were devastated. I knew Jerry was having a real hard time with this news and he took it out on all of us.

Jerry got some horrible news in '92; his mom was dying of cancer. He became determined to be in the Mr. Wisconsin Contest, I think more for his Mom than himself. I think he needed to show her he was okay and that he would be a success at anything he said he could do. That year, Jerry, with the help of a trainer and a lot of patience from his family, got into the best shape of his life. He could barely walk after his intense training sessions and his mood was less than desirable, but he got into the Mr. Wisconsin Contest. We were so proud of him, that day he shined. If you didn't know it, you wouldn't have been able to tell that his hip was bad. He and his trainer were able to come up with a routine that didn't compromise Jerry's chance at winning. His mom was there and we all watched in amazement as Jerry took 3rd place, a feat that we all thought was pretty monumental. A guy with a bad wheel, taking 3rd place over younger, healthier men. We were all very proud.

That, I believe was the last great time we had with Jerry, attitude wise, until after his hip replacement. His mom died in '94 and that seemed to aggravate the already debilitating hip problem. He was hard to live with, always defensive. He even made our family trip to Disney World somewhat miserable, he couldn't tolerate all the walking, so we had to leave him by the pool at the hotel.

Well, the day finally came when Jerry's body finally got the best of him. He had a hernia that needed to be repaired, so in January of 1997 he surgery to repair the hernia. It had to be done before the hip could be done. That went pretty well, so in March of '97, he was scheduled for hip replacement. He was very nervous and crabby. He made life interesting.

The hip replacement went great, but the Sciatic Nerve was aggravated from the surgery. Jerry became a nightmare to live with. He was out of work almost eight months and that was mentally draining to all of us especially Jerry. It took some time for everything to re-adjust itself in Jerry, but when it finally did, everything was wonderful.

Jerry became a human being again. Our relationship got much better. He started riding his bike again and now shares that with our son. He's a whole person again, the guy I knew and loved before. That hip replacement has made a definite change in my life and my kid's lives. Jerry is a happy, healthy, caring, loving and energetic man again. Now we can enjoy the time spent together.

# CHAPTER TWELVE:
## Interviews with Hip Replacement Patients

This chapter is dedicated to fellow hip replacement patients. A chance for you to hear some patient's stories about what this surgery did for them. Here they are.

SUSAN B'S STORY:
(77 years old when she had it done)

When Jerry asked me to write how I felt about the experience of the hip replacement, I was happy to share my experience with him. I was diagnosed with Osteoarthritis when I was 60 years old. At that time, I was very active. I loved to play golf and take walks down by the lake front. As time went on in my early 70s, I was not doing as much as I wanted to. My life style changed from one of pretty active to one of almost total inactivity, because of the degeneration of my right hip. I decided to go see a doctor about my options. I was skeptical and scared to even consider a surgery to replace my hip. At my age, I was not sure what to expect. It would have been nice to talk to someone that had gone through it or at least someone's account of their experience. I could no longer take the pain. The pain had taken my life from me and when I learned there was a chance to get it back I needed to do it. I had the surgery and almost immediately the pain in my hip was gone. It was almost like a miracle, the pain I had felt for 15 years or so was all of a sudden gone. I had a long road to recovery, but I was determined to hit the lynx someday again. I wanted to so bad, that I made it my goal. I am proud to say I'm back playing golf today and going for walks by the lake as well. I want you to know that if I could get through this, anyone can. Good luck with the book Jerry, and may anyone whom decides to have this surgery have a successful one and get their life back as well.

TOM C.'S STORY:
(47 years old when he had it done)

I am a construction worker, have been all my life. I have been fortunate in business and cannot complain. But there was a time that one incident I had changed my life for a while at least. I was working on a job site and was walking on a bar of steel waiting for a crane to lower me some materials for the job I had to do, one thing led to another and the next thing I know, I was falling two stories down luckily on some sand and gravel, not cement. The fall left me with a broken left hip and shoulder. I was in pretty bad shape for awhile, but eventually everything healed with what I thought was okay. I thought I was lucky. Well, a year or so after, my shoulder was fine, my hip was getting worse, I needed to see a doctor about my options. It seems the crack in my socket made the joint sloppy, which caused the bone to move around too much causing the cartilage to deteriorate. He recommended a total hip replacement. How I'm a firm believer in God gave you stuff you need body wise, why would I think about putting fake things in my body. I'll tell you why. I couldn't take the pain anymore. If the doctor told me there was a 10% chance I would be better I would have taken those odds. I went ahead and had the surgery. I came out of it smelling like a rose. A short period of rehabilitation and before I knew it I was back on the job site—what I call good as new. Thanks to modern technology, and thanks to God getting my life back in order.

ANOTHER STORY:

I would like to tell a more recent story. I used to golf. My degenerating hip did not allow me to turn on the ball perfect. Every time I swung hard on the ball it pained me immensely. I could no longer enjoy the game of golf for other reasons than just a bad score. It seems a great golfer; maybe the greatest of all time had this same predicament recently, caused him to miss the first Masters in his 30 or 40 years, Jack Nicholas. His hip was bad enough he went ahead and had a total hip replacement. His surgery too allowed him to get his life back, and actually his livelihood—his profession as a golfer. I recently saw him coming out of the hospital after the surgery on the T.V. and not long after that I think two months or so, he was back on T.V., this time in a golf tournament. I just wanted to make sure all of you whom read this book gets the Big picture and take everything into account when deciding your own fate in relation to the hip.

## GLEN H'S STORY:

I had the pleasure of meeting a very fine gentleman in the locker room in the club that I belong to the other day. I noticed the scar on the side of his hip just about the time he noticed mine. We kind of had a laugh together and began conversing about our situations. It seems we both had similar situations which stemmed from a deterioration of the hip joint. The thing we didn't have in common was our ages. He was 89 and I was 37. This just goes to show you that there is no limit age wise as far as I am concerned to look into a hip replacement. He stated that his quality of life was not good anymore. Even at age 89, things can be done to your ailing hip joint, to get your life back to normal. What a wonderful feeling.

# CHAPTER THIRTEEN:
## My Present Condition as of the End of the First Hip Replacement

This chapter was written after my rehabilitation period following my first hip replacement back in '97. I will pick up my life leading up to, during and after my second hip replacement in the second part of this book.

My status as far as my physical disposition is one of very stable, and strong. Every day I thank the good Lord for loving me and blessing me with this new found physical happiness. I must tell you, the saying: God helps those who help themselves, is also true. You must be prepared to work at getting better. You must be driven to succeed in your rehabilitation. The part God will help you with if you trust him, is the times you run into real blocks along the way. I guarantee the rehabilitation road will have its bumps, it is pertinent for you, and the individual to stay focused on the goal of achieving physical independence. The way you eventually aspire to be: physically normal.

I have had the good fortune of progressing physically by leaps and bounds. One big reason is I am totally focused and driven. A positive mental attitude (PMA) is necessary to succeed in anything in life for that matter.

You need not concern yourself with negative thoughts or negative people. Don't let anyone tell you it can't be done with talk like "This is the best you'll ever get," or anything like that. How many times have you heard that someone who was supposed to have had terminal cancer and given no hope to live, have turned it around to be totally cancer or disease free; A miracle, yes totally unforeseen. Probably not in the patients mind, chances are that individual willed the cancer away with positive thought and a lot of prayers. On the other hand, I have heard stories on the opposite end. Stories where an individual went in for a routine check up and a couple months later were dead. Fate, maybe, but I've seen situations where given the news, that particular individual just sort of gave up, let their mind become filled with negativity where there was almost no chance for them to conquer the problem. So reiterate a PMA is very, very important and necessary when you go into this type of surgery. It is major surgery and should be treated as such. It is going to change your life in a major way.

I am now training with weights as I had when I was 20 years old. I have slowly worked my way back into working on my legs. I have recently leg pressed over 500 pounds. Something I will not recommend to anyone. I have methodically set myself up for a successful outcome from this major surgery I have gone through. My hope is that you or someone you know will have the same results. You must know your limitations as well. There are limits with your new hip. There are no ligaments or tendons holding your hip in place. The scar tissue around the hip and strong muscles around the hip joint help to hold the joint in place and sturdy as it can be. Putting yourself in stressful situations concerning your hip will only jeopardize your condition. Use your head when it comes to physical activities. My doctor informed me he did not want me to run a marathon or even run for an extended period of time. No off road bicycling, or rigid sports.

I can, however, do most anything else virtually pain free, thanks to Doc Wood, God, and the surgery!

# CHAPTER FOURTEEN:
## Facing the Financial Responsibilities of a Major Surgery

This chapter is dedicated to the financial aspect of a total hip replacement. Financial responsibility would probably be one of or the most important things that would prohibit or rather keep someone from being able to have a hip replacement done; besides, of course, just plain being afraid of having it done. Fortunately, for the human race, the improvements the medical field has made in the last 50 years have enabled people with chronic pain or a deadly disease, to be able to have options to allow them to live longer, better lives. I call what was done to me a modern day medical miracle. Unfortunately, today miracles do not come cheap.

The rising cost of health care today is a very big issue. Most politicians have to address healthcare plans they intend to pursue to lessen the burden financially on the average everyday citizen. The cost of health care as a whole today has gotten out of control. It's almost as bad as the salaries of professional athletes.

I guess I can sympathize with people in the medical profession justifying the money they make. I'm sure the attitude of some medical field professionals is if people have money enough to pay exorbitant ticket prices to accommodate salaries of professional athletes that play games kids play, then people certainly would pay anything to have an opportunity or chance of changing their lives for the better, or even save their life by paying for an operation or medicine. You would think that as a society, professionals that are involved daily in saving and changing lives for the better should far out wage a professional athlete that plays games for a living. Wouldn't you think?

Unfortunately, that is not the case. We, as a society, have put far too much emphasis on sports personalities and the importance of playing games. Something has to happen to bring things around to a legitimate medium. Until then the cost of everything keeps rising including the cost of health care. Therefore, it is in everyone's best interest to make sure they prepare financially for a rainy day. You've heard the saying, when it rains it pours. I was in the middle of a week long monsoon, with no umbrella, when it came time for me to face up to the possibility of having to get a new hip.

I had no idea how much a new hip would cost, that is, where my first advice to whomever needs to have it done comes in. Get an estimate! Yes, just like body work at an automobile shop.

Be familiar with your health insurance let them know what type of procedure you are going to have. How long of a hospital stay is predicted, what's covered, what's not. Do not guess or assume anything—KNOW IT FOR A FACT!

It is a good thing for most people especially if they are the head of the house hold, major "bread" winner or sole bread winner and or athletically active to get disability insurance. It's too late to purchase a policy once you are hurt. Some policies cover your home mortgage, truck or car payments, etc… An ounce of prevention is worth a pound of cure. Be prepared. My operations, a total left hip replacement, cost approximately $100,000.00 three years ago. Between my insurance, which is pretty decent, and my wife's insurance, which is also decent, not a lot had to come out of my pocket, as far as the operation was concerned. *But*—I did not have disability insurance; I was naïve. I did not get hurt at work; I did not receive workman's compensation. All I received while I was off was a disability insurance check that my local union estimates as a benefit. This check helped, but it didn't even cover groceries for a week for my family of five. I'm not complaining. I was not schooled in setting up myself financially to handle being out of work for what turned out to be five months between my hernia and my hip.

I put some figures to the whole thing—between lost gross wages as a pressman, savings account depletions and a loan to help me; we absorbed a $50,000.00 loss. Wow, was that a serious setback!

But you know what? I was miserable before the surgery, I would have figuratively given anything for my life back…and I'd do it again.

My father and my in-laws helped us out a bit. And three years later we recovered most of the loss. And I'm me again.

Please, take my advice in this chapter. I have a little true story to tell you.

I had been playing football with some buddies of mine about 20 years ago. I caught a pass, made a cut, and went down. I tore some cartilage in my knee. It was pretty sore, and I remember someone referring me to a doctor whom had done work on him. I did not know he was the doctor of a couple of professional sports teams. I also did not know enough to get an estimate and find out what was covered by my insurance and what was not. Turns out since he was a doctor of some professional sports team his prices were twice what most other doctors was! What does that mean? It meant not only was I responsible for 20% of the cost of a normal and customary charge for an arthroscopic knee surgery because my insurance covered 80% of a normal and customary charge of that surgery, but because he charged double because he was "the Man," I had to pay for what turned out to be a whole another surgery to boot. Example: hypothetically speaking, an arthroscopic knee surgery would customarily cost $2,000.00. My insurance would cover $1,600.00, I would pay $400.00.

Since "hot shot" doctor charges $4,000.00—my insurance still only covered $1,600.00, because "hot shot's" charge was twice the industry standard, I had to pay $2,400.00! That sucked! So please, don't you be "suckered." Educate yourself. Become familiar with your insurance agent, your policies, possible policies beforehand, and the cost of your particular surgery. You'll be sorry if you don't. Unfortunately, I speak from experience...

Check it out.

# CHAPTER FIFTEEN:
## The Fear Factor

It is human nature to feel uneasy, skeptical, and just plain afraid of things we know nothing about. The feeling of uneasiness while contemplating a major surgery is even more intensified. The whole idea of replacing something God gave me from birth, with something fabricated by man is what kept me from having my hip replacement. The way I felt the last couple years before my surgery should have pushed my surgery up that couple of years, but the bottom line is, I was scared. The possibilities of bad side effects, dislocation, blood clots, infection, etc…of my particular surgery, scared the hell out of me. The thing that pushed me over the edge to finally having it done was the pain in my hip joint was so bad I didn't care about anything anymore…the thought of even dying did not concern me.

The human brain is a very complex organ and your mind can play tricks on you. There were times when I would try to convince myself that my hip pain was not that bad, and sometimes that line of thought would make me feel better…I think? There was finally no way around, or out of the constant pain. That was my pressure point, the point of no returns. I was ready to do whatever it took to alleviate my pain. I was lucky; there was some thing that could be done. I had options. Some people don't. Some people live with chronic pain their whole life, because there's nothing they can do about it. Either their physician has not pin pointed the cause of the pain, or the pain is caused by some thing not treatable, etc. That is when the individual either learns to cope with the pain themselves or they go to a pain clinic. Those are the options. If nothing can be done, deal with it, or deal with it!

In closing, I was a fool to put off a surgery that could have alleviated my pain. I had a way to rid myself of my pain, and chose to put it off as long as I could. In retrospect, I should have had the surgery done a couple of years before I did. I hope from now on I will not hesitate or procrastinate when something bothers me physically, but human nature says I probably will.

# CHAPTER SIXTEEN:
## Final Thoughts About the
## First Hip Replacement Experience

The purpose of this book was to give you not only my story of how I was before the surgery and how I am now, but also give you some technical background on what happens in the surgery and what to expect after the surgery. I also have touched a bit on some downside possibilities of the surgery, as well. I have not dwelled on these points so as to stay away from as many negatives as possible. A big part of this whole thing is that you have a good possibility of getting your life back.

I am doing, very, very, well right now. I am two years plus after the surgery. I have a weight lifting partner and we are training very diligently. My family life is very good as well most of my pleasant disposition is back. I didn't have much to begin with, I'm sure my family would say, but my attitude health wise is the best it's been in many years.

When I see people now that have hip problems, I feel their pain. I want to, and have approached people and preached to them there is something that can be done to change that. Almost like a "Born Again." I know God had a hand in the success of my surgery and I know he's had a hand in having me write this book. I am preaching the good word that with the success of a hip replacement there is an opportunity to have a new life. A life free of hip pain and of normal walking I know I am not the only one that this has had a positive effect on, and you've heard some of these stories.

There is one gentleman in particular I am showing concern for. He lives in my community. I have told him I will introduce him to my doctor, sit with him before surgery, help him with the rehabilitation, and I mean it. I'm not quite sure why, but I would love for him to get his life back. He was a great athlete in his younger days. I think he is going to take me up on my offer. I know if he does he will have a great possibility of having a new hip and a new life.

Thank you for reading this book so far and I hope if you know somebody that is like this or you are like this, believe me when I say it can change your life. Tell them about this book and have them read it, it just might change their life! Please read on about my second hip replacement.

THE END
of Hip Replacement #I.

Now for Volume II:
The Right Hip Needs Replacing
June 2006

# VOLUME II
# HIP REPLACEMENT
## #2

# CHAPTER SEVENTEEN:
## Hip Replacement #2
## June 2006

My life was going along fairly well for some 10 years o so after my first hip replacement. I had competed in two more body building contests placing in the top two in both. My right hip was showing some discomfort the past few years but nothing I was too worried about. I took a position at my work as a lead pressman on a very big printing press, an 8-color Komori. I call it the "Beast of Burton." It is very physically demanding to work on this particular press. My left hip replacement handles the rigors of my daily routine rather well. Guys that work on the press with two good hips feel the aches and pains daily. Over the holidays of 2005, Christmas and New Years, my wife and I went bowling with her brother and his wife. We had a great time that night, but I remember waking up the next morning with a very sharp pain in my right hip, one that would not go away. Back in '93 when I first saw Doctor Wood for my arthritic hips, both hips were bad. The left hip was worse than the right, but I told Doc Wood to take them both out. He said it was absurd to even suggest that. After the first replacement I knew it would just be a matter of time before I would need the right hip done.

Fortunately, there was a 10 year span between the two. But now that the right hip was bad, I have to confess I tried to convince myself that it wasn't that bad I guess it's human nature.

My daughter was finishing plans for her upcoming wedding. The ceremony was to be held in August. I was looking forward to it, but my hip was getting sorer by the week. It was now March 2006. Everyone, including myself, was worried about my ailing hip, and possibly not being able to walk my daughter down the aisle. The decision to have my hip replaced was wearing on me. The thought of going through all that surgery and rehabilitation again was looming large and heavy on my mind. The days were going by and eventually my hip started to lock up on me, something my other hip never did. I would sit down and try to get up, not being able to, without a ton of pain and agony. It felt like there was a spot in my joint that would not allow the hip to move. Like it was locked, it is some of the most excruciating pain you could imagine. I remember the last straw was getting to work one morning and taking 20 minutes to get to stand up. That was it, I had decided to schedule my replacement as soon as I could, so I could rehabilitate before the wedding and be able to properly walk my daughter down the aisle. I would need 3 months for all of that, so bring on Doc Wood again, for another miracle. My second hip replacement.

# CHAPTER EIGHTEEN:
## Another Visit to Aspen Orthopedics and Super Surgeon Doctor James Wood, M.D.

The phone call was made. I was scheduled to see my pal Doc Wood, at Aspen Orthopedics. The anticipation of seeing the good doctor was bitter sweet. I was looking forward to seeing him and how he was doing. I was hoping he was happy to see me as well, but not under the circumstances. He walked into the waiting room where I was. He had a big smile on his face, I was sure happy to see him again. He is such a nice guy, and he had changed my life for the better some 10 years ago. We made small talk and got down to business. X-Rays first, then we'd talk some more. I waited. X-Rays came back not really showing much. I said tell my hip that. I wondered how that was possible. The Doctor didn't doubt what I was complaining about but he needed a more in depth look. He scheduled a CAT-scan, said we would talk after the results got back. I went in for the "routine scan". No big deal...right? That's what I thought. I was wrong. It turned out to be a half an hour of complete hell. I was told to lie flat, motionless in the tube with nothing under my knees, while the scanner took pictures of my hips. My right hip hurt so bad in the position, it locked up, and I couldn't believe the pain. I had tears in my eyes, and did not last the entire half an hour. I had to abort after 20 minutes, but they got all the information they needed. It took me another 10 minutes to sit up from that position. It was time to schedule the replacement.

# CHAPTER NINETEEN:
## Hip Replacement #2
## Finally Scheduled
## June 2006

I have to admit to everyone that I had to eat my own words of advice. The bit about not putting off a procedure medically that could change your life for the better, even after I proved it to myself, by going through it first hand. The skepticism was fresh in my mind, though. The thought of going through all that surgery stuff; Rehabilitation, the possible down side of things, possible infection, dislocation, blood clots, etc... All the uncertainty of everything, AGAIN! Would it be worth it? You bet it would. I can tell you from first hand experience for the second time around, it was all worth it. I will, however, for everyone's benefit, go through everything associated with the experience, some similar, some very different. Stay with me, the second story is every bit entertaining as the first...

Doctor Wood met with me to discuss the scan results. He agreed I needed a new hip. I knew it before the scan. Anyhow, we agreed on a date. Surgery was set for June 17, 2006. I was happy and apprehensive. I had a vivid recollection of what was directly ahead of me. I thought I was ready for it. The second go around, strap it on, psych up, I could handle it, I had been through it before, and came out on top! I was already ahead of the game; I didn't have to deal with the sciatic nerve or back problem like last time. This should be a cake walk right? That wasn't really the case, although I don't think it ever got as bad as some of the stuff I dealt with the first time around.

# CHAPTER TWENTY:
## Getting Prepared for Round 2

My preparation for hip #2 was no different than the first. I had to go down to the blood center to give my own blood in case I needed some. I had to go to the hospital to have blood drawn for tests they need. I had to see my family doctor for a pre-op physical, to make sure I was in good enough shape to withstand the surgical impact on the body. All the things I had to do turned out well. I was on my way for my June date with destiny.

I will say that truth be told, if I hadn't had a time restraint on me to make a decision on the surgery, I probably would have put it off. My daughter's wedding was putting a lot of pressure on my decision. A lot of people were counting on me to be in good shape by wedding time. I know some people reading this are probably thinking what's wrong with me. Been through it successfully once, it's a no-brainer. Have it done and suck it up. Nothing has ever been that easy for me. Besides, it's major surgery. Now that I am writing the last of the book, I can honestly say its life altering just going through it all. I'm not sure I want to go though another hip replacement, ever. It is undoubtedly two of the most stressful situations of my life. Yes, I could not have gone through the rest of my life with either of the hips I was born with. I remember a couple months after surgery #2, Doc Wood said that if I had come to see him in an earlier life, say in the 60's, with the same hip discomfort, the medical field could not have done much for me. He said they would have probably given me a bunch of pain meds, a walker, crutches or even a wheel chair. Why would I not want to go through another one? Because it's scary, the unknown, will it go alright? Will I survive the surgery again, etc., etc., etc...

# CHAPTER TWENTY-ONE:
## Surgery Day Is Finally Here for Hip #2

Once again the night before surgery was somewhat sleepless, just like 10 years ago. My wife and got up in the morning with not a lot of talking. I was pretty tense. The trip to the hospital was again both too long and too short. I stopped by the admitting desk and checked in. My brother-in-law Jimmy Kaz met my wife and me there. He got to see us only to say good luck and that he loved me…I love Jim, probably more than he knows. He's my brother-*in-law*—minus the in-law…I love him like a brother, he is a good man and he has always been there for me. We went to the pre-op room to get prepped for surgery. You pretty much wait around in that room, small talk with your wife. It's the room before the next waiting room. It's the last point where your loved ones can be with you. Next stop is where they start your I.V. I was on my way there before I knew it. Got settled in my curtain area, and waited for everything to happen. I.V. gets set up, anesthesiologist visits with you, and then the doctor says hi and asks how you're doing. My particular surgeon has been a God sent to me. He showers up with a big smile on his face, told me everything was going to be ok, and gave me a hug. I can heart felt say I love him too; much like my brother-in-law or a father who loves a son. He is a great man in my eyes, and a great surgeon. My family and I are grateful for him and what he does. He is a tribute to his profession. He is what all medical students should aspire to be. I mean this with all my heart. Thank you Doctor James Wood, M.D.

# CHAPTER TWENTY-TWO:
## My Diary from the Second Surgery Stay at the Hospital

I remember waking up from surgery a bit groggy. I got my senses about me much like the first hip, and like the first time as the seconds went by the pain got so intense I almost started screaming. Not the hip, but the surrounding area, the buttocks, and the upper thigh—all of almost everything hurt or seemed like it did—all at once. I'm not sure if the doctors or nurses purposely back off on the pain medication so the patient can come out of the anesthesia. I'm not suggesting that this is even a possibility, but if it were, I would understand. When I expressed my displeasure of how good I felt, the nurse instantly gave me a shot of pain meds and I instantly began to feel better. I was the Mr. Chatty Patty. They couldn't shut me up. Everybody was my best friend. Not a care in the world. I felt if we were all at a bar I would be buying the drinks.

I will say having spent way too much time in recovery rooms the nurses that work in that room are some of the nicest people in the world. They monitored my vitals for the next hour or so, until everything stabilized enough to move me to my room for the next 5 days or so. When I got to the room some of my loved ones were there waiting to see me. It sure is nice to be loved. I really don't show how much I appreciate my loved ones enough and don't realize how much they love me until I saw the worry and concern in their faces. It's something you can't fake. When something bad happens in my family—We try to divide the pain among all of us. It seems to help. My support group did just that while I was in the hospital.

First day over all was ok—nothing way up or way down. Pretty even keel, for a while.

I am the first to admit I am not the greatest patient. That is an understatement if you asked the nurses that tended to me this go around. In fact, one nurse called me Mister Happy! I don't remember being this cautious about moving around in and out of bed the first time. I don't know why, but sitting up in bed to swing my legs over the side and move to a chair was totally freaking me out. The first three days I was a basket case. I was telling all of the nurses, all three shifts, how to properly care for me. Where to stand, when I was getting up, how to move my legs, how to do just about everything, until one particular nurse had enough. She scolded me and I took it. She went on about; did I think I was the first hip replacement patient they had ever cared for? She said, "My God! This is the orthopedic floor. Chill out." Let them do what they were trained and being paid to do. She was very professional and nice about everything. From that point I was much better. Well I was better, I think.

I got a feeling of anxiety when I would reposition myself from lying in bed to sitting in a chair by the bed. It took so much energy, physical and mental that I would stay in the new position way too long. So long, that I was so sore that I wouldn't want to move again, not good.

Pain meds in proper circumstances and applications are a heaven sent. The medication they had me on made life the first few days bearable. They helped me be able to move around and do some of the exercises necessary for the recovery process to happen. There was a new pain creeping in the picture, and it wasn't my back. It was a sharp pain behind my knee cap, not bad enough to complain about…yet!

The third day was supposed to be better than day two. Unfortunately, that wasn't the case. The pain in my knee was consuming my thoughts. Doctor Wood was gone and unavailable for the weekend until Monday. I had an "on call" doctor. I met her, she was very nice. I told her of my knee cap pain, by this time it was killing me, I think that's how I put it.

She proceeded to tell me that she was sorry my knee hurt. She continued by explaining to me what they did in surgery that might account for the pain in my knee. Big time details about how they bent my leg behind me and off to the side to dislocate the hip—then they broke the hip socket and on and on…you get the picture. At least I did, and about that time I felt like throwing up.

Let it be known my hip was not the issue, my glut that was cut to get at the hip and of course my knee—overall the doctor visit, and all of day three sucked!

Day 4 started with more of the same. Moving from the bed to the chair, using my walker and crutches. Walking with my therapist; telling her my concerns about the pain in my knee. I thought it might be a blood clot or maybe my knee cap was broke. In comes Doc Wood, I'm all over him, like a sticky booger. I'm going a mile a minute; he can't get a word in edgewise. Finally, he says it couldn't be a blood clot, it's in a soft tissue area, and if I wanted he would x-ray my knee. I wanted!

It turns out, nothing wrong on the x-ray—no blood clot, but I was still dealing with the pain. With Day 5 right around the corner, the possibility of going home should have made me happy. I still couldn't put pressure on my knee. Try and sleep tonight, it will be better tomorrow?

Going home, no matter what the circumstances, is always a good thing. This day was no different. I was happy to be going home. I did, however, suggest they cut my leg off at the knee before I left. Honest to God! Instead they fit me with a full leg immobilizer—from my upper thigh to my ankle. That did the trick. I could put pressure on my leg now without going through the roof! I was on my way home before I knew it. I couldn't help but pray the worst was behind me while my wife drove me home. I was feeling anxious and anxiety about getting home. My four dogs were a concern. I love them and they love me. They get so excited to see me everyday when I get home from work. I was worried about them jumping up on me after being away for almost a week. When I got home it's as if they knew not to jump. They sensed something was wrong with dad. I love those four pups. As I got settled in my favorite chair I couldn't help but feel a bit relieved and yet a lot overwhelmed with the long road to recovery ahead of me. I wish all I had to do was follow the yellow brick road!

# CHAPTER TWENTY-THREE:
## The Time from
## Second Surgery Until Now

Directly after surgery, the very next day home my knee cap started feeling better. I don't know exactly why or how, but I think it was from moving around more then I had been. I started by doing my exercises religiously & maybe that dislodged something behind the knee cap. All I know is I was very happy it was feeling better. This next story is going to be hard to believe, but it's the truth. Swear to God!

Later in the first week of being home from surgery, I ordered a big dumpster. Yes, a very big garbage dumpster. For what you ask? We have a very nice above ground oval pool. We had been kicking around the idea of tearing apart some of the wood deck surrounding the pool. You guessed it. I made sure to be careful, took my time, and slowly and methodically with the help of my youngest daughter, disassembled most of the wood deck. We had hammers, screwdrivers and a sawzall. In less than *ONE* week out of surgery I took on a task that would have been a lot for a normal guy. We had that dumpster filled in ten days! The lord is my Judge; ask my family and my neighbors. I think this is worthy of being on Ripley's Believe It or Not. Probably not the smartest thing to do, but I did it. I don't know what drives me to do the things I do, but I knew I did not want to just sit around and do nothing. I am what most would call an "excessive compulsive." What my wife loves about me, is what she hates about me. There's no middle ground. It's all or nothing with me. It's just the way God made me. It keeps me constantly challenging me, gives me purpose.

Three weeks after starting the demolition project I was finished and looking for something else to do. This would send my doctor into a fit, so don't you try doing what I did directly after surgery. I was lucky nothing bad happened. In fact, I know it was pretty stupid. I did, however, plan my every step while doing it.

I remember watching the NBA finals between the Miami heat and Dallas Mavericks. I don't normally watch T.V. in the evenings, but I actually enjoyed watching all 7 games. I had my wife, who was awesome, set up a bachelor pad on the first floor of our house. That was very convenient. I did look forward to sleeping with her as soon as I could.

My four dogs kept me plenty of company day and night. I had visitors most every day. One particular visitor besides the obvious (relatives and close friends) was a very nice lady whom had just gone through her hip replacement. A friend of a dear friend, she had heard I had just gotten out of the hospital and was taking visitors. She was actually still walking with the aid of a cane and still on her rehabilitation trail. I was excited to see her as I let her in. We talked about the ups and downs of each others surgeries and in the end wished each other well. She was slowly walking away towards her car with her cane shaking her head in disbelief. Before she left I told her about my demolition project. It was he third month after her surgery. I could only look at her and hope my time of recovery would be less. One of the biggest reasons, was there was an upcoming project at work that I wanted to be part of. I stuck my neck out before surgery in the pre-planning stages and said we could do it a certain way.

I felt I needed to follow it through 'til fruition and back up what I said. I dedicated myself to push hard enough in rehabilitation, that I could indeed return to work instead of 3 months, what turned out to be 2 months. Not only did I have to be in shape enough to go up and down stairs and dress myself, but work shape, busting my tail on the "Beast of Burton" the 8-color Komori press. That, I thought, was kind of amazing.

I want everyone to know, if they are contemplating having a hip replacement, it's not easy. You have to set realistic goals to make the surgery a success. I understood going into the surgery, what was in store for me after having been through it before. I was very focused and that's why both off my surgeries were successful.

I successfully returned 100% full duty to work two months after surgery. No light duty anything, full throttle ahead. My fellow co-workers, whom I have the utmost respect for, and myself not only put together a very successful project, but we won "Best of Show" at an awards banquet for Midwest Printing Companies. We won Best of Show for a catalog on Cruiser Boats 2006. The project lasted three weeks, grueling, not only mentally, but physically as well. I managed to get through it all by staying focused, watching what I was doing and praying as well. I am most proud of that moment. Winning that award made me feel more of a professional pressman that years gone. What I had to overcome to achieve that was very rewarding. I am a printer. It's what I do for a living. It's what puts food on my family's table, and a roof over our heads. I was happy to have a goal to get back to work as soon as I could, because I enjoy what I do!

Next up for me was my oldest daughter's wedding. Getting back to work was first, back in the swing of things, then focus on successfully walking my daughter down the aisle.

The wedding was beautiful. Probably, the most beautiful wedding I'd ever been to. The fact that I was participating in full force as the bride's father was a tribute to the job Doctor Wood did, the marvel of modern day medical procedures and my God blessed sense of dedication to getting better.

I cannot put into words just how blessed I am to have been the recipient of 2 prosthetic hips, Bi-lateral Hip Replacements, as doc would put it. When I see the x-rays of my prosthetic hips I come to tears. The reality of seeing all that metal is jaw dropping. I listened to the restrictions the good doctor was laying on me for the second time around and couldn't help but feel fortunate to have all the pain of my ailing hips gone. I am, however, subject to having a somewhat fragile immune system. Infections are not a good thing or are they something or take lightly, whether it's an infected tooth, a cut, a scrape of a knee or a thorn in the thigh. This next story is a bit scary, at least it was for me...

I had successfully come back to work, glowingly walked my daughter down the aisle, and now hunting season was fast approaching. I am an avid bow hunter. I love matching wits with the whitetail deer. I love whitetail deer so much that I took up a second profession to preserve the whitetails my clients harvested. I am a taxidermist and artist for the past 25 years. To say the least I was glad all the hip stuff was behind me and I could concentrate on hunting. It was October my favorite time of year.

This particular hunting trip I was on, had me accompanied by my best friend Rod and my brother-in-law, Jim. We were bow hunting on a 40 acre parcel of land I owned up in Adams County, Wisconsin. Hunting in early November—"The Rut." The only time of year the deer are in reproduction frenzy. Big bucks throwing caution to the wind looking for a chance to hook up with a mate. What could go wrong?

The first evening hunt was incredible. I saw 9 different bucks, 5 worthy of putting on the wall. While on the stand I remember feeling a bit queasy. I had chills, light headedness and felt sick. Earlier in the week I got a cut on my upper thigh, looking for a doe I harvested while bow hunting back home. In the stand I felt a decent size lump on my thigh. It itched, and felt a bit sore. Over the weekend the lump got to be softball size. Monday morning I went to work and made it 2 hours before I asked to call my doctor, Doc Wood.

I called him and told him I might or rather, probably had an infection in my upper thigh. He did not hesitate to clear a spot to see me immediately. He saw me, took one look at the lump and said this is very serious; I could lose my leg, my hip, and possibly my life! WOW! Was I scared? You betcha!

The next two days were a blur. Before I knew it, the next day I was admitted to the hospital for emergency surgery to extract the infection.

One week later I got out of the hospital with a softball size hole in my upper thigh. I had escaped disaster by less than 1 inch. If the infection had gotten down to my spike (femur) in my leg, I probably would have lost my leg. Less than 1 inch came between the infection and my leg. God loves me.

I spent the next seven weeks recovering from the infection. I had to have an infection suction device on the wound 24-7. Seven weeks later I had the device taken off and my wound closed up. Doctor Wood has changed my life twice, and now saved it once. What else could he do for me? I owe this man more than I could ever repay. He's a special guy and I love him like a father.

2006 was both great and terrible for me. I am blessed; I am sitting at my kitchen table finishing up my book. A book I hope inspires people who are on the bubble, so to speak; undecided on whether or not to have a hip replacement.

I am living proof bad things happen to good people, genetically, self inflicted, contracted/contagious, etc... I am also proof good things can come out of bad. I'm living the dream. Somebody asked me if I could come back in another life who would I come back as? I said without hesitation...ME! I love my life. It's good to be me. God loves me and I thank Him everyday. I've been blessed and lucky. I've had the benefit of having the best orthopedic surgeon work on me, a loving family and a good attitude... all of which are necessary to come out of a hip replacement with a smile.

Research a reputable surgeon, do your part in preparing for your surgery once you, your surgeon and your family all agree that's what is the best thing for you is! Stay in as good a shape physically as you can. Eat well and stay positive. Ask God to walk with you and watch over all of which is to be.

I hope with all my heart that this book touches a lot of people. I've spent a lot of time writing it with hopes of convincing at least one person that there is an option to dealing with bad hips. You can have them replaced. No, it's not a walk in the park but it's not a terrible journey. It's what you make of it.

Good luck and remember, God is up there and He's there for all of us, at least I think so. Lean on Him and you'll get through your hip problems maybe some day to be able to say with me...

HIP-HIP HOORAY!

# CHAPTER TWENTY-FOUR:
## An Overview of What to Do and Not to Do After Surgery

Also,
A Pictorial View of the Exercises That Helped Me in Recovery & Rehabilitating My Body

- DO NOT move your operated hip toward your chest (flexion) any more than a right angle, 90°
- DO NOT sit on chairs without arms.
- DO grasp chair arms to help you rise safely to a standing position. Place extra pillows or cushions in your chair so that you do not bend your hip more than 90°
- DO NOT bend both knees to get up. Keep operated leg straight and in front while getting up.
- DO use a chair with arms. Place your operated leg in front and your off leg well under.
- DO NOT sit low on a toilet or chair.
- DO get up from a toilet as directed by your therapist. Use

the elevated toilet seat if you have one…you should.

- DO NOT bend all the way over.
- DO NOT turn your knee cap inward when sitting, standing, or lying down.
- DO NOT try to put on your own shoes or stockings in the usual way. By doing this improperly you could bend or cross your operated leg too far.
- DO follow your therapist's advice on ALL activities.
- DO NOT cross your operated leg across the midline of your body.
- DO NOT lie without a pillow between your legs.
- DO keep a pillow between your legs when you roll onto your good side. This will keep your operated leg from passing midline.

LAYING SIDE KNEE BENDS:
Laying on your side, keeping your involved leg away from your straight flat leg,
Slowly raise your knee to your abs. Not past 90°. Then slowly straighten leg out.
3 sets, 10-15 reps. Good movement for outer thigh and abs.


BUTTOCKS WALK:
Clear a path on the floor. Sitting up legs flat on the floor. Much like an inch worm, inching himself across the floor. Raise one but cheek a few inches, use you heel of the off leg to grab an inch or two of floor and in a waddling motion move back and forth inch by inch across the floor and then back. It works the stiffness and soreness out of your butt! Feels Good.


LAYING SIDE LEG RAISES:
Laying on your side, take a pillow and put it between your legs. Take involved leg and raise it slowly about 10-15 inches. Hold for 5 seconds, slowly lower, relax. Repeat. Later on, in rehab, try not relaxing at the completion and keep going. You'll feel a burn. That's a good thing. Shows the exercise is working. No pain, no gain. Each leg, 3 sets, 10-15 reps.


KNEELING LEG KICKBACKS:
While kneeling on one leg, slowly take involved leg backward until it's straight. Slowly bring leg forward to a 90° angle again,

and back and forth, etc.. (3 set, each leg, 10-15 reps.) This is a good exercise for strengthening your glut—abs., hamstrings, etc...

## LAYING ON STOMACH—SINGLE LEG RAISES, REVERSE STYLE:

Keeping your upper torso flat on the floor and one leg flat on the floor, slowly raise the involved leg backwards as far as you can. Slowly lower and relax. Work up to 3 sets, 10-15 reps, this strengthens the glut and hamstring.

## STENGTHENING EXERCISED QUADICEPS SETTINGS:

Propping your feet up with a pillow or towel, tighten the muscles on the top of your thigh. At the same time push the back of your knee downward into the bed. The result should be straightening your legs. Hold for 5 seconds, relax 5 seconds. Progress to 20 reps, 3 times a day..

## ACTIVE ABDUCTION:

Place a smooth surface (cad table, plywood sheet, etc...) under your legs. Begin with your legs together, and then spread them apart as far as you can. Hold them apart for 5 seconds. Return to starting position. Progress to 20 reps, 3 times a day.

ACTIVE INTERNAL AND EXTERNAL ROTATION:
Begin with your legs straight and a comfortable distance apart.
Roll your legs inward so that your kneecaps are facing each
other. Hold for 5 seconds. Roll your legs outward and hold for
5 seconds. Progress to 20 reps, 3 times a day.

ACTIVE HIP AND KNEE FLEXION:
Lying on your back with legs straight, toes pointed toward the
ceiling; arms by your side. Keeping the heel in contact with the
bed, bend your hip and knee. Return to starting position.
Progress to 20 reps, 3 times a day.

GLUTEAL SETTING:
Lie either on your back or on your stomach with your legs
straight and in contact with the bed. Tighten your buttocks in a
pinching manner and hold the isometric contraction for 5
seconds, relax 5 seconds. Progress to 20 reps, 3 times a day.

ISOMETRIC HIP ABDUCTION:
Keeping your legs straight, together, and in contact with the
bed, place a loop o belt around your thighs and attempt to
spread your legs. Hold the contraction for 5 seconds, relax 5
seconds. Progress to 20 reps, 3 times a day.

## KNEELING STRAIGHT LEG RAISES:
This movement will strengthen your buttocks. It will be sore at first. The glut is cut during surgery to get at the actual hip joint. You need to grit your teeth and work through the pain. It is a very good movement to strengthen that whole area.

\* NOTE: This movement would be performed after you have done,
>    1. Gluteal settings and
>    2. Isometric hip abductions, that I explained earlier

## BENT KNEE SINGLE LEG RAISES:
This is also a good, "first up after surgery" movement. Keeping your "off leg" bent, slowly raise your opposite leg, keeping the involved leg straight. Tighten the glut (buttocks) as you lower the leg. Slow is the key.
3 sets each leg, 10-15 reps.

## LYING LEG LIFTS (STRAIGHT LEG):
A good exercise for strengthening the abdominal muscles as well as quadriceps—the top part of the leg.
START SLOW! Slowly raise your straight legs up about 12-15 inches off the floor. Slowly let them down. Work your self up to 3 sets, 12-15 repetitions.

SQUAT:
This exercise is called a squat. It is a movement that power lifters do with heave weights. The rehabilitating patient will do well by just doing the squat with their own body weight. Once again, leaning up against a wall to start is best.
Start with short movements at first. Slowly working your way up to the full squat. 3 sets, 12-15 reps. This movement will build up your gluts, thighs, lower back and hamstrings. A very good "core" building exercise.

Here is a very good exercise to strengthen the glut (buttocks) and the front of the leg (quad) . Start by leaning against the wall to stabilize yourself. Balancing on 1 leg, probably not a good idea.
Start by slowly lifting your leg to 90° angle. Directly after surgery, be happy to just lift your leg. Work yourself up to 3 sets of 8 reps each leg.

Do not pass mid point with your knee. My doctor said he would be amazed if he could not hear me scream if I dislocated my hip by doing this. Believe me—I focused every minute of everyday to not pass my knee past mid point. You should too!

This is definitely a NO-NO! This position puts the affected hip in serious jeopardy of being dislocated. A lady I referenced in a part of the book, that dislocated her hip by trying to paint her toenails, was probably close to sitting in this position—not good! Be smart.

This is another photo of how to properly get up from a sitting position. The couch we had was firm, but I elected not to sit in it until I could properly get up without my crutches. If all you have is a couch to sit in, prop yourself up with a bunch of pillows to not allow yourself to sink below the 90° angle.

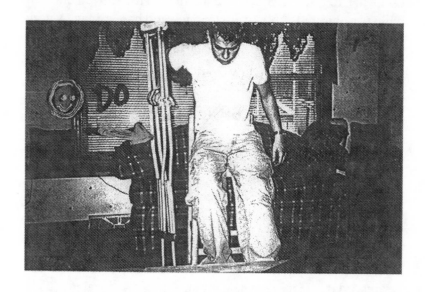

Notice the barstool type chair my son is getting up from. He elected not to sit in the couch behind the chair, good move for the recovering patient. Also, notice he is using his crutches (my crutches) to aid in his rise up from the stool. This is the proper way to get up from a sitting position while rehabbing.

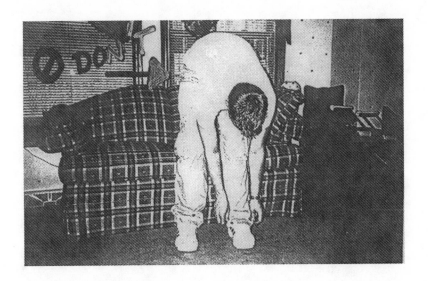

Do not bend over to tie your shoes...until your doctor says. While convalescing have someone else tie your shoes or use slip-ons. This posture would surely lead to prosthetic dislocation.

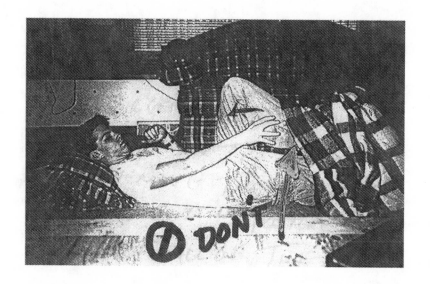

DO NOT pick up your blanket with your operated leg. You might risk bringing the knee up past the 90° angle. Besides it's an unstable movement. Well planned & deliberate movements are the best way to ensure not doing something stupid or ill advised.

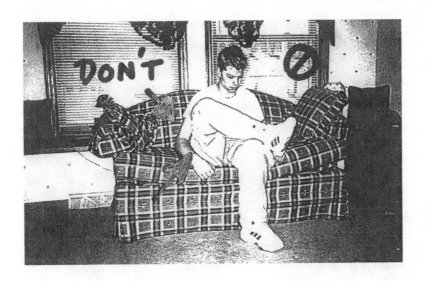

DO NOT ever pick your operated leg up in this position, especially directly after surgery. I don't recommend sitting like this even years after surgery. Reason being—scar tissue basically holds the hip in place along with strengthening the muscles surrounding the hip. This sitting posture jeopardizes the strength of all of that.

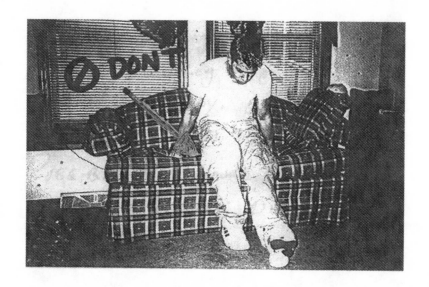

First point of this picture is the couch. After surgery you do not want to sit on a low sinking type of chair at all. You want to prop yourselves higher up—almost like a bar stool. You want to guard against going past the 90° angle with your body. The second point of the "don't" is notice there is no crutch or walker to aid in getting up from the sitting position. Always have your walking aids near by.

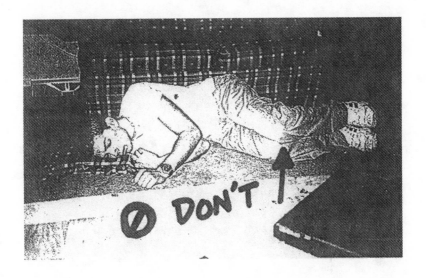

DO NOT lie on your side without a pillow between your legs. This pillow will not allow your leg to cross over mid point of your body. Without the pillow between your legs, there is a good possibility of your leg crossing over mid point & possible dislocation of the new joints.

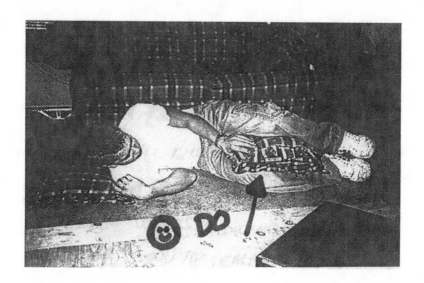

This IS the proper way to lie in the fetal position which feels the best after surgery. Notice the pillow between my son's legs. This is very important. It will not allow your knee to cross mid-point of your body...pass mid-point with your knee—risk dislocation of hip!
PERIOD!

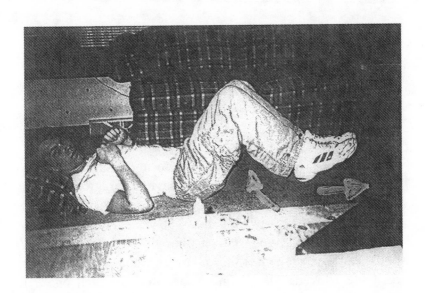

LYING KNEE RAISES:
Lying flat on your back, slowly raise your knees up towards your lower abs. Lower your knees back to a straight leg position.
This will build up your lower abs and give your legs a decent "flexion" movement to get all the juices flowing. A very good movement, early in rehabilitation. 3 sets, 10-15 reps.

# CHAPTER TWENTY-FIVE:
## Family—My Salvation

I have dedicated the last chapter to my family and close friends. Without them, I would not have made it through the surgeries as successfully as I did.

I will start with my wife of almost 30 years. I think she must have invented the saying "you only hurt the ones you love". All of the stuff she's put up with from me over the years, she must really feel loved. All kidding aside, we love each other. I remember coming home from the hospital after surgery #2, she had the whole first floor set up for me, the patient. She set up a bed the living room, so I wouldn't have to climb the stair to our room. My walker was standing next to the bed to help me get in and out safely. The powder room was set up just for me, raised toilet seat and all my necessary toiletries. The refrigerator and cupboards were filled with my favorites. And of course, all my pups were waiting to console me. The only thing missing was "Clarence and the ringing bells from" It's A Wonderful Life". I am truly blessed to have Lynn; I am ashamed that sometimes I loose sight of that.

Next: my children. Somehow I've always been driven to want to leave my mark on this world. This book means a lot to me, a sort of legacy. When I look at my true legacy, it is my children. God chose me and Lynn to raise the three beautiful children we have, trying to keep bad things from happening to them. I've spent more than a few sleepless nights worrying about them, letting them stumble and fall and being there to pick up the pieces. They all have grown up to be such interesting and caring people. I know this because they were such a help to me when I was down. I love m kids very much, I think they know it.

My siblings are next. First, my older sister, Carie. If you saw us together, you'd know from one look that we are related. And if you heard us out together having a good time, even if you didn't see us, just by hearing us, you'd know we are related. Most people kiddingly say that Carie is a female Jerry (me). I cannot deny any of it and wouldn't! I love my sister; we grew up in a household with challenges and we got to be very close. She has a big heart; she remembers everyone's special days and sends cards to everyone, a real sweetheart. We periodically get together with her and her husband Jim to go out dancing and partying, we always have a great time. Before I started having trouble with my hips, I was a lot of fun "cutting a rug" with her and my wife. As the pain in my hip increased, the fun was cut in half. I would try to get through the pain, but I would pay dearly the next week, the limping and the stiffness. Finally it got to the point where I didn't even want to go anymore. It was sad. The silver lining, after both surgeries and rehab, I'm back to "cutting a rug" again. My sister has always been there for me and that will never change. I will always love Carie, Jim and their sons Kenny and Cody; I have been blessed to have them in my life.

Last but not least, my little brother Doug. We have been through a lot over the years. He was there for me after my first surgery, a source of humor for me when I was down, he always could cheer me up. We had a special connection; we could share thoughts with just a look. Life takes some weird turns. I've always thought I could control whatever life dealt me, I was wrong. Things sometimes change and you don't understand why, that's where my brother and I are at now. I will always love him, no matter what and I hope he's happy. I'm still the only one who can make fun of him!

My in-laws Frank and Ann Marie McLeod deserve special mention. They are two of the nicest people I have ever had the pleasure to be associated with. I love them both very much; they are like parents to me. They have been there for me and my family. Their unconditional love for their entire family is amazing to me. I hope to be as successful as them, they lead by example. Frank and Ann Marie are truly heaven sent and I am touched by the way they have loved us all.

All of my in-laws are a loving, supportive force; I thank God for having all of them in my life.

I also have some terrific friends, I am very fortunate. Three of my best buddies, John, Rod and Dan were a source of strength for me when I was struggling to get back on my feet after the surgeries. I am grateful to everyone in my life; it's the support of friends and family that push you to success.

This is very important, to those of you who decided to have the surgery; your support group is probably the most important part of rehabilitation. Having encouragement and help around you while you recover is very beneficial to a successful recovery. As the song goes," Lean on me, when you're not strong, I'll be your friend, and I'll help you carry on"…